AF756980

Appendicitis - Current Insights

Edited by Vanita Ahuja and Ayaka Tsutsumi

Published in London, United Kingdom

Appendicitis - Current Insights
http://dx.doi.org/10.5772/intechopen.1002568
Edited by Vanita Ahuja and Ayaka Tsutsumi

Contributors
Aaron Rodwell, Adelais K. Tzortzopoulou, Ajith Kumar Sankarankutty, Anas Shikha, Asem Kasem, Dylan Gracias, Hesham Sayed Ahmad, Ishith Seth, Jorge Elias Junior, José Sebastião dos Santos, Karamveer Singh, Leonardo Resende Sousa, Lokadolalu K. R. Shanbhogue, Lyndel Hewitt, Marcos Antônio Marton Filho, Mekki Hassan, Mohamed Alfatih Hamza, Navin Kumar, Rafael Kemp, Ricardo Ribeiro Correa Filho, Somprakas Basu, Summi Karn, Zafir Babiker

© The Editor(s) and the Author(s) 2025

The rights of the editor(s) and the author(s) have been asserted in accordance with the Copyright, Designs and Patents Act 1988. All rights to the book as a whole are reserved by INTECHOPEN LIMITED. The book as a whole (compilation) cannot be reproduced, distributed or used for commercial or non-commercial purposes without INTECHOPEN LIMITED's written permission. Enquiries concerning the use of the book should be directed to INTECHOPEN LIMITED rights and permissions department (permissions@intechopen.com).

Violations are liable to prosecution under the governing Copyright Law.

Individual chapters of this publication are distributed under the terms of the Creative Commons Attribution 4.0 License which permits commercial use, distribution and reproduction of the individual chapters, provided the original author(s) and source publication are appropriately acknowledged. If so indicated, certain images may not be included under the Creative Commons license. In such cases users will need to obtain permission from the license holder to reproduce the material. More details and guidelines concerning content reuse and adaptation can be found at http://www.intechopen.com/copyright-policy.html.

Notice

Statements and opinions expressed in the chapters are these of the individual contributors and not necessarily those of the editors or publisher. No responsibility is accepted for the accuracy of information contained in the published chapters. The publisher assumes no responsibility for any damage or injury to persons or property arising out of the use of any materials, instructions, methods or ideas contained in the book.

First published in London, United Kingdom, 2025 by IntechOpen
IntechOpen is the global imprint of INTECHOPEN LIMITED, registered in England and Wales, registration number: 11086078, 167-169 Great Portland Street, London, W1W 5PF, United Kingdom

For EU product safety concerns: IN TECH d.o.o., Prolaz Marije Krucifikse Kozulić 3, 51000 Rijeka, Croatia, info@intechopen.com or visit our website at intechopen.com.

British Library Cataloguing-in-Publication Data
A catalogue record for this book is available from the British Library

Appendicitis - Current Insights
Edited by Vanita Ahuja and Ayaka Tsutsumi
p. cm.
Print ISBN 978-1-83634-251-9
Online ISBN 978-1-83634-250-2
eBook (PDF) ISBN 978-1-83634-252-6

If disposing of this product, please recycle the paper responsibly.

We are IntechOpen, the world's leading publisher of Open Access books

Built by scientists, for scientists

7,500+
Open access books available

196,000+
International authors and editors

215M+
Downloads

156
Countries delivered to

Our authors are among the
Top 1%
most cited scientists

12.2%
Contributors from top 500 universities

WEB OF SCIENCE™

Selection of our books indexed in the Book Citation Index
in Web of Science™ Core Collection (BKCI)

Interested in publishing with us?
Contact book.department@intechopen.com

Numbers displayed above are based on latest data collected.
For more information visit www.intechopen.com

Meet the editors

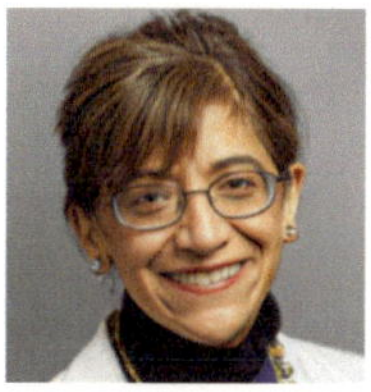

Vanita Ahuja, MD, is a dedicated educator, surgeon and researcher. With a rich background in surgery and training, she is a devoted leader committed to serving veterans. As a veteran herself, Dr. Ahuja began her medical journey in the US Navy, attending the Uniformed Services University of the Health Sciences. She completed her surgical internship at Portsmouth Naval Medical Center and served in Japan and Guam, where she was the Chief Medical Officer on board the USS Frank Cable. Dr. Ahuja then completed her general surgery residency at Johns Hopkins Hospital and earned both her MPH and MBA from Johns Hopkins. Dr. Ahuja has also played a significant role in training surgical residents as a program director. Most recently, she served as the Chief of General Surgery at the Connecticut Healthcare System-Veterans Affairs and was an Associate Professor of Surgery at Yale School of Medicine. She is a Fellow of the American College of Surgeons and has served as a Consultant for the American Board of Surgery.

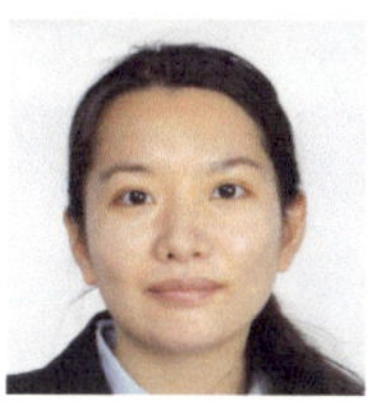

Ayaka Tsutsumi, MD, is a dedicated clinical researcher with experience in leading medical institutions. She previously served as a Research Associate at Yale University School of Medicine and is currently a Research Fellow at SSM Health Cardinal Glennon Children's Hospital. Her work focuses on advancing clinical research, with a special interest in integrating artificial intelligence into surgical practice to enhance patient outcomes and surgical precision.

Contents

Preface

Appendicitis, an age-old affliction, continues to be a formidable presence in surgical practice worldwide. Despite our medical advancements, its prevalence underscores the enduring importance of understanding and effectively managing this common pathology. However, the landscape of appendicitis care has undergone a remarkable transformation in recent years.

We have witnessed the dawn of minimally invasive surgical techniques, revolutionizing the patient experience by enabling same-day operations and significantly reducing recovery times. While disruptive, the global pandemic, COVID-19, inadvertently accelerated research into non-surgical treatment options, offering a potential paradigm shift in our approach to appendicitis. Furthermore, the burgeoning field of artificial intelligence has begun to permeate the diagnostic and therapeutic realms, promising to refine and optimize our strategies for managing this condition.

Yet, amidst these advancements, a stark reality persists. Access to quality healthcare remains a privilege, not a universal right. For those residing in rural areas of developing countries, the journey to essential medical care can be arduous and often involves hours of travel. This disparity in access creates a world of differences in patient outcomes. Within these pages, you will encounter a testimonial that offers a poignant glimpse into this reality. This perspective will undoubtedly challenge and broaden the understanding of Western readers.

This book aims to provide a comprehensive and up-to-date picture of appendicitis, encompassing its diagnosis and treatment across both pediatric and adult populations. We attempted to synthesize the latest research, clinical insights, and technological advancements while acknowledging the diverse realities of healthcare access worldwide. We hope this work will serve as a valuable resource for clinicians, researchers, and anyone seeking a deeper understanding of this ubiquitous surgical challenge.

Of note, the views expressed in this book are those of the authors and do not necessarily reflect the position or policy of the Department of Veterans Affairs or the United States government.

Vanita Ahuja MD, MPH, MBA, FACS
Associate Professor of Surgery,
Yale School of Medicine,
New Haven, Connecticut, USA

Ayaka Tsutsumi
Research Fellow,
SSM Health Cardinal Glennon Children's Hospital,
St. Louis, Missouri, USA

Section 1

Adult Appendicitis

Chapter 1

The Effect of COVID-19 Lockdown on Appendicitis Severity and Management

Aaron Rodwell, Dylan Gracias, Ishith Seth and Lyndel Hewitt

Abstract

The COVID-19 pandemic placed substantial strains on healthcare systems globally causing downstream sequalae on emergency surgical conditions including acute appendicitis. The primary aims of this study were to examine rates of complicated appendicitis, conservatively managed uncomplicated appendicitis and outcomes of acute appendicitis management before, during and after the New South Wales' COVID-19 lockdown in Australia. Retrospective analysis of patients with acute appendicitis in a NSW local health district between 4th December 2019 and 13th October 2020 was undertaken. Patients were grouped temporally into Pre-lockdown, Lockdown or Post-lockdown groups. No significant change in the rates of complicated appendicitis during the lockdown compared to periods immediately before and after the lockdown were found. Patients with complicated appendicitis tended to be older and have longer hospital stays. Conservatively treated uncomplicated appendicitis rates did not increase during the lockdown period. The findings indicate potential for lower threshold for investigation and management of suspected acute appendicitis in older people and criteria for conservative management of uncomplicated appendicitis may require revision. Analysis of pandemic surgical rates could enhance bed management planning for future disasters, ensuring optimal patient safety. Further research is required to delineate the effect of lockdowns on acute appendicitis and may inform changes to practice.

Keywords: lockdown, complicated appendicitis (CA), COVID-19 pandemic, appendicitis, conservative treatment

1. Introduction

1.1 Level of evidence: III

Acute appendicitis refers to acute inflammation of the appendix, proposed to be most typically secondary to appendicular lumen outflow obstruction [1]. It is a common intra-abdominal surgical emergency with an individual lifetime incidence of 7–8% [2, 3]. Acute appendicitis presentations are typically classified into uncomplicated appendicitis and complicated appendicitis [3]. Uncomplicated appendicitis

IntechOpen

(UA) is defined as a simple phlegmonous inflamed appendix, whilst complicated appendicitis (CA) includes appendicitis complicated by rupture, peritonitis, gangrene or abscess [4]. The diagnostic distinction between CA and UA is usually made by radiological imaging or diagnostic laparoscopy [5].

The differentiation between complicated and uncomplicated appendicitis is vital to determine specific management principles of each appendicitis case. In particular, it guides the need and urgency of surgery, can inform the intraoperative process as well as the postoperative management [4]. Uncomplicated appendicitis (UA) is primarily managed surgically by appendectomy or, for select patients, via conservative antibiotic therapy which carries an inherent 25–41% 90-day failure rate depending on presence of appendicolith [6, 7]. CA on the other hand is managed by surgical means in appropriate candidates with the operative technique varying depending on the subtype of CA and patient factors [8]. The class of appendicitis also has a direct impact on postoperative outcomes, with CA correlating with increased mortality rates and length of hospital stay [3]. Furthermore, CA confers a greater healthcare burden and cost associated with the increased length of stays and the defining complications needing further management [9].

One of the major contributors to acute appendicitis progression to CA is time until intervention [10]. Many factors can impact how rapidly health care services are accessed by patients suffering from acute appendicitis. These include but are not limited to, geographic, environmental, sociocultural and socioeconomic factors [11, 12]. During the recent Coronavirus Disease (COVID-19) pandemic, the strain on healthcare systems globally may have influenced CA rates because of patient's reluctance to present to hospitals, healthcare staffing issues, hospital policies and protocols, resources and the delivery of medical care [13–15]. These factors could potentially delay time to treatment thereby impacting CA rates during the pandemic.

A 2021 systematic review and meta-analysis conducted by Köhler et al., which included 21 international studies, reported an overall reduction in the incidence of acute appendicitis, an overall increase in CA rates (26.6% compared to 22.2%, OR 2.00, $p < 0.0001$, $I^2 = 72\%$) during the pandemic as well as increased rates of conservative antibiotic only treatment as the management of choice for acute UA [16]. These findings are in contrast to studies conducted in Denmark, Switzerland, Iran, Taiwan and Italy which found no statistically significant difference in CA rates during the COVID-19 pandemic [12, 17–20]. In fact, Jantzen et al. found a non-significant reduction in CA incidence during the Denmark nationwide lockdowns for which they postulated a reduction in infectious disease transmission as an explanation [12]. Despite this, the majority of recent studies conducted in Israel, Argentina, Switzerland, Lithuania, Turkey, Italy, the Republic of Korea, Taiwan, USA, and the Netherlands, found statistically significant rises in rates of CA during the COVID-19 pandemic [9, 21–29]. These increases varied from 1.22 fold to 4.245 fold [23, 28]. These variations could be due to differences in healthcare systems, as well as political and public factors. In Australia, few studies have been conducted analysing the impact of the pandemic on acute appendicitis, with conflicting results [30–32]. There is currently insufficient evidence demonstrating a conclusive or consistent link between the pandemic and its effect on acute appendicitis.

Whilst much of the current literature found an increase in the rates of CA during the COVID-19 pandemic it is important to note that there was heterogeneity in terms of study design, sample size, follow-up periods, degrees of COVID restrictions, and

DOI: http://dx.doi.org/10.5772/intechopen.1008160

healthcare systems. The lack of consistent findings highlights the need for further studies to investigate the effects of the COVID-19 pandemic on the rates of CA. Furthermore, there is limited literature describing the rates of CA, conservative management of UA and resultant outcomes during the times before and after lockdown periods.

2. Methods

This study aimed to analyse acute appendicitis presentations in a NSW-based local health district during the COVID-19 lockdown period. This period was defined by the NSW State Government's stay-at-home orders in the Greater Sydney region, and presentations during this time were compared to equal periods immediately before (pre-lockdown), and after (post-lockdown). Three patient groups were made based on these time periods. Specifically, we aimed:

1. To determine the impact of the COVID-19 lockdown in NSW/Greater Sydney on the rates of acute appendicitis presentations among adult patients in Illawarra Shoalhaven Local Health District (ISLHD) hospitals.

2. To examine the clinical characteristics and outcomes of patients with acute appendicitis, including the rates of complicated appendicitis, in-hospital mortality, length of hospital stay, and all-cause 28-day readmission across the different periods.

3. To analyse the relationship between age and gender concerning acute appendicitis presentations, including potential age-related trends in complicated appendicitis and gender-related differences within study groups.

4. To investigate the rates of conservative treatment for uncomplicated appendicitis and assess the readmission rates for patients managed conservatively, including any differences between the study groups.

A retrospective cohort study was conducted using routinely collected de-identified data from a New South Wales based local health district. This study was approved by the local Ethics Committee, UOW & ISLHD Health and Medical Human Research Ethics Committee Project ID: 2022/ETH01792.

The routinely collected de-identified data was made available from the Illawarra Shoalhaven Local Health District. These data are a sub study of a larger project being led by Dr. Chantal Campbell titled 'Antibiotic vs. Surgical Management of Uncomplicated Acute Appendicitis in the Illawarra Shoalhaven Health District: a 20-year retrospective analysis comparing proportions and trends in management, 28-day readmissions, and length of stay (ISLHD/LNR/2021-147).

The retrospective analysis included data from all patients, aged 18 and over, who presented to an emergency department within the local health district, and were diagnosed with acute appendicitis during the defined pandemic periods. Participants were allocated to one of three groups: the lockdown group – defined as the 105-day NSW/Greater Sydney lockdown period from 18th of March 2020 to 30th of June 2020; the pre-lockdown group from 4th December 2019 to 17th March 2020; and the post-lockdown group from 1st July 2020 to 13th October 2020. The three resultant groups each had a 105-day period.

Data for patients were included in the different groups based on time of hospital presentation for acute appendicitis. The NSW/Greater Sydney lockdown period used in this study was defined based on NSW State Government's order of allowing no more than 100-person indoor gatherings. Other restrictions were variable but included restrictions on leaving place of residence without reasonable excuse, social distancing measures of 1.5 metres, limitations on indoor and outdoor public gatherings (limited to two people at its most strict), non-essential travel bans and aged care visitation restrictions. It should be noted that during the lockdown period restrictions on indoor gatherings were at times more restricting than only allowing 100-person indoor gatherings. Patients that presented within one group but were readmitted outside of the dates forming that group were included in their original group only.

The severity of appendicitis was classified according to ICD-10-AM (The International Statistical Classification of Diseases and Related Health Problems, Tenth Revision, Australian Modification) codes used for hospital admissions and SNOMED-CT® AU (Systemized Nomenclature of Medicine – Clinical Terms Australian Extension) used in Emergency Department presentations:

- Codes used for uncomplicated appendicitis:
  - ICD 10 AM – K35, K35.8, K36, K37, K38.9 [33]
  - SNOMED-CT® AU -72,048,003, 235,769,005, 196,785,005 [34]
- Codes used for Complicated appendicitis:
  - ICD 10 AM – K35.1, K35.2, K38.1 [33]
  - SNOMED-CT® AU -62,224,002, 266,439,004, 28,845,006, 51,036,000, 196,781,001, 64,252,005, 4,998,000, 286,967,008, 47,693,006, 95,547,004 [34]

Non-acute appendicitis codes were excluded, and some of the codes above were included but deemed to be contentious; K38.9, K36, K38.1, 196,785,005 [33, 34]. These were contentious as some of the included patients may not have had acute appendicitis. Data was collected based on the diagnosis of acute appendicitis without consideration of patient comorbidities or concurrent pathologies, and hence patients with concurrent colorectal cancer or inflammatory bowel disease for example, including their management were not specified. Similarly, pregnant females while included in this study, were not specified.

Surgical treatment was defined as patients who had either an open or laparoscopic appendicectomy and patients not having these surgeries were deemed to have had conservative treatment mainly consisting of antibiotics, analgesia with clinical and biochemical monitoring. Of note, robotic appendicectomy was not available at any of the hospitals studied. Access to emergency operating theatres was still readily available during lockdown as was anaesthesia availability, however this was not statistically examined.

Statistical analysis was performed using *jamovi* Version 2.3 [35] Continuous variables were described using means and standard deviations or medians and ranges if data were asymmetrical; categorical variables were described using counts and percentages. Categorical variables between three groups were compared using the Pearson's chi-square test. Independent *t*-tests were used to compare continuous variables between two groups, and one-way analysis of variance (ANOVA) was used to compare continuous variables across three groups. A p value of <0.05 was deemed statistically significant.

3. Results

A total of 452 adult patients presented to the hospitals with acute appendicitis during the three study periods. This included 131 patients in the lockdown group, 163 patients in the pre-lockdown group and 158 patients in the post-lockdown group (**Figure 1**). This depicts a decrease in acute appendicitis presentations in the lockdown group.

There was no statistically significant difference in age or sex distribution between the three groups (**Table 1**). Rates of complicated appendicitis among the three groups showed no statistically significant difference (**Table 1**). However, as depicted in **Figure 2**, the proportion of complicated appendicitis was higher in the post-lockdown

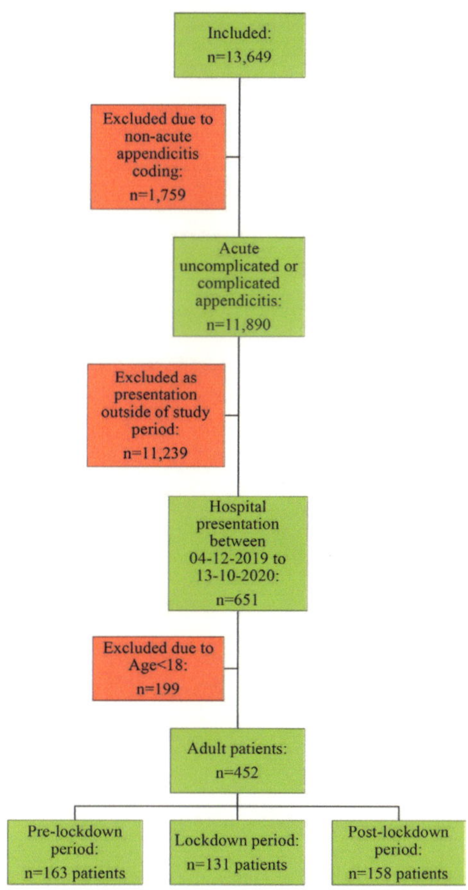

Figure 1.
Study Population included in the pre-lockdown period, lockdown period and post-lockdown period.

	Total	Pre-lockdown	Lockdown	Post-lockdown	p-value
	n = 452	n = 163	n = 131	n = 158	
Age, mean (SD)		37.48 (17.25)	40.79 (18.21)	38.82 (16.33)	p = 0.285
Sex					p = 0.630
Male, n (%)	224 (49.56)	76 (46.63)	68 (51.91)	80 (50.63)	
Female, n (%)	228 (50.44)	87 (53.37)	63 (48.09)	78 (49.37)	
Classification					p = 0.345
Complicated, n (%)	116 (25.66)	38 (23.31)	31 (23.66)	47 (29.75)	
Uncomplicated, n (%)	336 (74.34)	125 (76.69)	100 (76.34)	111 (70.25)	
Treatment modality					p = 0.102
Surgical, n	427	149	126	152	
Conservative, n (%)	25 (5.53)	14 (8.59)	5 (3.82)	6	
Hospital Stay					
Length of Stay, mean (SD)		2.99 (2.42)	3.19 (2.05)	3.69 (7.38)	p = 0.455
28-day readmission, n (%)	8 (1.77)	5 (3.07)	3 (2.29)	0	p = 0.099
Mortality	0	0	0	0	

*SD – standard deviation.
†*Appendicitis Classification, Sex, Treatment modality and 28-day readmission were analysed by Chi-square testing.*
‡*Age, and LOS (length of stay) differences were analysed using one-way ANOVA.*
§*Statistically significant findings (p < 0.05) are shown in* **bold.**

Table 1.
Patient demographics, length of stay, treatment modality and mortality of acute appendicitis patients during the COVID-19 pandemic.

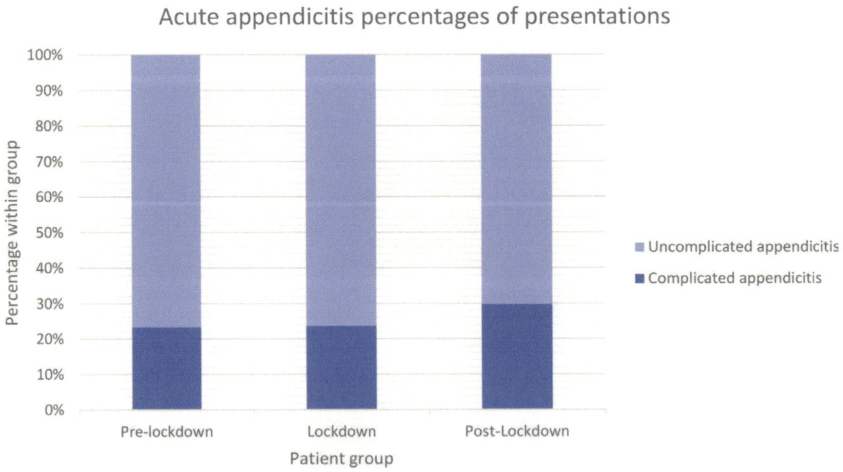

Figure 2.
100% Bar chart of patient percentages by category of appendicitis in the pre-lockdown, lockdown and post-lockdown periods.

	Pre-lockdown			Lockdown			Post-lockdown			Overall		
	CA n = 38	UA n = 125	p-value	CA n = 31	UA n = 100	p-value	CA n = 47	UA n = 111	p-value	CA n = 116	UA n = 336	p-value
Age, mean (SD)	41.18 (18.27)	36.35 (16.84)	p = 0.131	51.00 (18.89)	37.63 (16.87)	**p < 0.001**	47.04 (18.70)	35.34 (13.90)	**p < 0.001**	46.18 (18.85)	36.40 (15.92)	**p < 0.001**
Gender			p = 0.917			p = 0.653			**p = 0.012**			p = 0.161
Male, n (%)	18	58		15	53		31	49		64	160	
Female, n	20	67		16	47		16	62		52	176	
Hospital stay												
LOS, mean (SD)	4.61(4.32)	2.50(1.01)	**p < 0.001**	5.00 (2.72)	2.63(1.40)	**p < 0.001**	6.62(13.07)	2.45(1.01)	**p = 0.001**	5.53(8.78)	2.52(1.14)	**p < 0.001**
28-day readmission, n	0	5	p = 0.210	0	3	p = 0.329	0	0		0	8	p = 0.094
Conservative management, n	3	11		0	5		2	4		5	20	

SD- Standard deviation, CA-complicated appendicitis, UA-uncomplicated appendicitis.
†Sex and 28-day readmission were analysed using a chi-square test. Age and LOS (length of stay) were analysed using an independent t-test.
‡Statistically significant findings ($p < 0.05$) are shown in **bold**.

Table 2.
Demographics, 28-day all-cause readmission and LOS among the three groups split by acute appendicitis classification.

group (29.7%) compared to the pre-lockdown (23.3%) and the lockdown (23.7%) groups (**Table 1**). As shown in **Table 1**, there was no recorded mortality among the patients who presented with appendicitis during the three study periods reviewed. A comparison of the three groups indicated that the length of stay was not statistically significantly different between them (**Table 1**). There was no statistically significant difference in the rates of all-cause 28-day readmission between the three groups (**Table 1**).

Complicated appendicitis patients were statistically significantly older in age than patients who had uncomplicated appendicitis during the examined period overall ($p < 0.001$) (**Table 2**), however this was not true for the pre-lockdown period group in isolation (**Table 2**). Although not explored further in this study, there was a statistically significant higher rate of CA in males compared to females in the post-lockdown period group ($p = 0.012$). There was a statistically significant longer LOS in complicated versus uncomplicated appendicitis patients overall and within each of the three groups ($p < 0.001$) (**Table 2**). There was no statistically significant difference in 28-day readmission between complicated and uncomplicated groups however, all eight 28-day readmissions were uncomplicated appendicitis patients (**Table 2**).

There were no statistically significant differences in rates of conservative treatment in uncomplicated appendicitis across the three groups (**Table 3**). Of the complicated appendicitis patients, there were three patients in the pre-lockdown group and two in the post-lockdown group that were managed conservatively. All 8 readmissions (5 in the pre-lockdown group, 3 in the lockdown group, 0 in the post-lockdown group) were from the 20 conservatively managed uncomplicated appendicitis patients which was of statistical significance ($p < 0.001$) (**Table 4**). As depicted in **Table 4**, readmission rates of uncomplicated appendicitis patients managed conservatively across the three groups were not statistically significant. LOS among UA patients did not differ significantly between the three groups.

	Pre-lockdown n = 125	**Lockdown n = 100**	**Post-lockdown n = 111**	**Total n = 336**	**X^2(df)**	**p-value**
Treatment type						
Conservative, n	11	5	4	20	3.07(2)	p = 0.216
observed % within group	8.8	5	3.6	5.95		
Hospital stay						
LOS, mean (SD)	2.50(1.01)	2.63(1.40)	2.45(1.01)	2.52 (1.14)		p = 0.569
28-day readmission, n	5	3	0	8	4.28(2)	p = 0.118
observed % within group	4	3	0	2.38		

**SD-standard deviation.*
†Treatment type was binomial, with surgical as control. LOS (length of stay) was analysed using ANOVA. 28-day readmission and treatment type were compared using chi-square tests.
‡Statistically significant findings ($p < 0.05$) are shown in **bold**.

Table 3.
Analysis of conservative treatment and readmission rate in patients with Uncomplicated appendicitis only.

	Conservative n = 20	Surgical n = 316	X^2(df)	p-value
28-day readmission, n	8	0	129(1)	**p < 0.001**
observed % within group	40	0		

*28-day readmission among treatment modalities was analysed using chi-squared test.
†Treatment modality was binomial, with surgical as control.
‡Statistically significant findings (p < 0.05) are shown in* **bold.**

Table 4.
Analysis of relationship between treatment modality and 28-day readmission in uncomplicated appendicitis patients only.

	Pre-lockdown n = 38	Lockdown n = 31	Post-Lockdown n = 47	Overall n = 116	p-value
Age, mean (SD)	41.18(18.27)	51(18.89)	47.04(18.70)	46.18(18.85)	p = 0.093
LOS, mean (SD)	4.61(4.32)	5.00(2.72)	6.62(13.07)	5.53(8.78)	p = 0.607

*SD – standard deviation.
†LOS (length of hospital stay) and age were compared using one-way ANOVA tests.
‡Statistically significant findings (p < 0.05) are shown in* **bold.**

Table 5.
Length of stay comparison in patients with complicated appendicitis.

There was no statistically significant difference in age or sex (data not shown) of complicated appendicitis patients across the three groups (**Table 5**). **Table 5** illustrates difference in LOS of complicated appendicitis patients was not statistically significant among the three groups.

4. Discussion

The study findings indicate that the COVID-19 lockdown in the Illawarra Shoalhaven Local Health District did not result in an increase in the rates of complicated appendicitis. These results align with prior research, including two small-scale Australian studies, which similarly found no statistically significant changes in CA rates during the pandemic compared to previous years [17–20, 31, 32]. However, this contrasts with a recent NSW-based study reporting higher CA rates in one local health district during the pandemic [30]. Several potential explanations for this discrepancy exist, including local health system's ability to maintain a low time to intervention during the lockdown, reduced transmission of infectious diseases during the lockdown that may precipitate acute appendicitis, and decreased emergency department presentations due to COVID-19 patient concerns. It is essential to acknowledge that limited research has explored the lockdown's effects, and our study did not compare CA rates to equivalent periods in previous years, potentially confounding results due to seasonal fluctuations [36].

In this study, all CA rates (23.3% pre-lockdown, 23.7% during lockdown, 29.7% post-lockdown) were either comparable to or lower than those reported in other pandemic-related literature [9, 16]. These lower rates are in contrast to those of an

American study which found that there were significant increases in CA (17.7% vs. 35.1%) during the pandemic, potentially due to patients not seeking appropriate, timely medical care [37]. However, it should be noted that this study was undertaken in USA which experienced a different COVID-19 climate and healthcare system to that of Australia.

This study observed that complicated appendicitis patients were more likely to be older than uncomplicated appendicitis patients, consistent with existing literature [38]. While the pre-lockdown CA patients were not significantly older than their uncomplicated appendicitis (UA) counterparts, this age difference emerged during the lockdown and post-lockdown periods. Possible factors contributing to these age-related trends may include reduced social contact, increased mask usage, enhanced hygiene practices, and lower viral transmission rates among younger individuals during lockdowns. This age-related trend persisted post-lockdown, indicating that the lockdowns' effects on appendicitis presentations might persist beyond the lockdown period as infection prevention strategies remain pertinent to individuals. However, the study did not specifically investigate the underlying reasons for these age-related differences, such as delayed presentation or reduced healthcare-seeking behaviour among older individuals, which would require further research [39, 40].

Unlike some prior literature, this study did not observe an increase in the rate of conservative treatment as the intervention of choice during the lockdown period [16]. Looking at international trends, conservative management was adopted more frequently in an attempt to reduce peri-operative mortality, infection spread, and hospital admissions at the time of healthcare system strain during the pandemic [16, 41–43]. This study's unique approach compared conservative management rates at different times around the pandemic, shedding light on the lockdown's specific impact on acute appendicitis management and outcomes. However, comparisons with previous years are necessary to provide a comprehensive understanding of the pandemic's effect on conservative management. Throughout the study period, the 28-day readmission, in-hospital mortality, conservative management, and CA rates did not significantly differ between the three groups. However, the study's limited sample sizes for conservatively managed disease and 28-day readmission rate should be noted before generalising these findings. The study's findings align with UK and US research supporting the safety and effectiveness of non-operative management of acute appendicitis in the short term [7, 44]. Nevertheless, a more comprehensive analysis comparing outcomes during a period in which change in management occurred is needed to determine if improvements are warranted.

Several limitations must be acknowledged, including the inclusion of contentious appendicitis codes, which may require case-by-case analysis in future studies. Additionally, the study did not examine confounding variables such as time to presentation, time to surgery, patient comorbidities, functional status and COVID-19 status, which may have widespread ramifications such as affecting CA rates, length of hospital stay, and having implications on the intervention chosen by healthcare practitioners. The study's narrow focus on one Local Health District and limited access to patient notes hindered comprehensive analysis, and future research should consider state-wide datasets and case-by-case analysis. The absence of comparisons with previous years limits our understanding of COVID-19's impact on appendicitis. Lastly, the small sample sizes for conservative management and readmission data reduce generalisability.

Future research should explore factors such as time from symptom onset to presentation, conservative management protocols, and COVID-19 effects on CA

DOI: http://dx.doi.org/10.5772/intechopen.1008160

rates in more detail. This study's strength lies in its examination of acute appendicitis throughout pre-lockdown, lockdown and post-lockdown periods, of which post-lockdown analysis was not undertaken by prior studies [9, 12, 45, 46].

While the study did not identify a significant change in CA rates during the lockdown, it is crucial to consider that our analysis was limited to one Local Health District and lacked comparisons with previous years. Therefore, further research is needed to determine if specific planning is required for future pandemics. Additional details regarding the numbers and demographics of individuals in need of surgical interventions could enhance bed management planning, particularly in anticipation of future disasters, to ensure an ongoing high standard of care throughout adverse situations. Additionally, the higher mean age of complicated appendicitis patients in this study suggests that planning for older surgical patients during future pandemics may be necessary. Given the higher healthcare system burden associated with CA patients, a lower threshold for investigations and interventions in older patients with suspected acute appendicitis should be considered. Further research, including age-specific analyses, could inform these measures. The absence of a statistically significant difference in length of stay between surgically and conservatively managed patients raises questions about the effectiveness of conservative management protocols, especially considering the much larger 28-day readmission rate observed. Hospitals may need to review their criteria for conservative management of acute appendicitis if the goal is to reduce the healthcare system burden while still maintaining an adequate level of patient care.

5. Conclusion

In conclusion, this study did not find an increase in the rates of complicated appendicitis during the NSW lockdown period. Higher mean age of complicated appendicitis patients compared to uncomplicated appendicitis patients was noted during and after the lockdown, warranting further investigation. Rates of conservative management of uncomplicated appendicitis did not increase during the lockdown period and length of hospital stay did not appear to differ between surgical and non-surgical management of uncomplicated acute appendicitis. Furthermore, all 28-day readmissions during the study were conservatively managed uncomplicated appendicitis patients. Future research should aim to provide a comprehensive understanding of these effects in order to guide clinical pathways in the event of future pandemics and by extension, future events that pressure our healthcare system.

Acknowledgements

Thank you to Professor Kate Curtis for approving use of the dataset and to Brendan McAlister and Stephen Moules for your help with data collection and cleaning. Thank you to Judy Mullan, Bridie Mullholland and the University of Wollongong Graduate School of Medicine for their guidance.

Conflicts of interest

No authors have any conflicts of interest to declare. No funding applicable.

Author details

Aaron Rodwell[1,2*], Dylan Gracias[3], Ishith Seth[4,5,6] and Lyndel Hewitt[1]

1 Department of Surgery, The Wollongong Hospital, New South Wales, Australia

2 Graduate School of Medicine, University of Wollongong, New South Wales, Australia

3 Department of Surgery, Townsville University Hospital, Queensland, Australia

4 Faculty of Science, Medicine, and Health, Monash University, Victoria, Australia

5 Department of Surgery, Peninsula Health, Melbourne, Victoria, Australia

6 Peninsula Clinical School, Central Clinical School at Monash University, The Alfred Centre, Melbourne, Victoria, Australia

*Address all correspondence to: aaron.rodwell@health.nsw.gov.au

IntechOpen

© 2024 The Author(s). Licensee IntechOpen. This chapter is distributed under the terms of the Creative Commons Attribution License (http://creativecommons.org/licenses/by/4.0), which permits unrestricted use, distribution, and reproduction in any medium, provided the original work is properly cited.

References

[1] Stringer MD. Acute appendicitis. Journal of Paediatrics and Child Health. 2017;**53**(11):1071-1076

[2] Bhangu A, Søreide K, Di Saverio S, Assarsson JH, Drake FT. Acute appendicitis: Modern understanding of pathogenesis, diagnosis, and management. The Lancet. 2015;**386**(10000):1278-1287

[3] Bowen J, Sheen J, Whitmore H, Wright C, Bowling K. Acute appendicitis in the COVID-19 era: A complicated situation? Annals of Medicine and Surgery. 2012;**2021**(67):102536-102536

[4] Mariage M, Sabbagh C, Grelpois G, Prevot F, Darmon I, Regimbeau J-M. Surgeon's definition of complicated appendicitis: A prospective video survey study. Euroasian Journal of Hepato-Gastroenterology. 2019;**9**(1):1-4

[5] Bom WJ, Scheijmans JC, Salminen P, Boermeester MA. Diagnosis of uncomplicated and complicated appendicitis in adults. Scandinavian Journal of Surgery. 2021;**110**(2):170-179

[6] Talan DA, Di Saverio S. Treatment of acute uncomplicated appendicitis. New England Journal of Medicine. 2021;**385**(12):1116-1123

[7] Collaborative C. A randomized trial comparing antibiotics with appendectomy for appendicitis. New England Journal of Medicine. 2020;**383**(20):1907-1919

[8] Sohn M, Agha A, Bremer S, Lehmann KS, Bormann M, Hochrein A. Surgical management of acute appendicitis in adults: A review of current techniques. International Journal of Surgery. 2017;**48**:232-239

[9] Petrauskas V, Poskus E, Luksaite-Lukste R, et al. Suspected and confirmed acute appendicitis during the COVID-19 pandemic: First and second quarantines—A prospective study. Frontiers in Surgery. 2022;**9**:896206

[10] Wonski S, Ranzenberger LR, Carter KR. Appendix imaging. In: StatPearls [Internet]. Treasure Island, FL: StatPearls Publishing; 2022

[11] Seqsaqa M, Rozeik AE, Khalifa M, Ashri HNA. Geographic influence on postoperative complications in children with complicated appendicitis: A single center study. Annals of Pediatric Surgery. 2021;**17**(1)

[12] Jantzen AT, Bang-Nielsen A, Bertelsen CA, Torp-Pedersen C, Kleif J. Incidence of appendicitis during COVID-19 lockdown: A nationwide population-based study. Scandinavian Journal of Surgery. 2022;**111**(2):14574969221089387

[13] Bersano A, Kraemer M, Touzé E, et al. Stroke care during the COVID-19 pandemic: Experience from three large European countries. European Journal of Neurology. 2020;**27**(9):1794-1800

[14] Blecher G, Blashki GA, Judkins S. Crisis as opportunity: How COVID-19 will reshape the Australian health system. The Medical Journal of Australia. 2020;**213**(5):196-198

[15] Kariya A, Krutsri C, Singhatas P, et al. Incidence of complicated appendicitis during the COVID-19 pandemic: A systematic review and meta-analysis. International Journal of Surgery Open. 2022;**45**:100512-100512

[16] Köhler F, Müller S, Hendricks A, et al. Changes in appendicitis treatment

during the COVID-19 pandemic–A systematic review and meta-analysis. International Journal of Surgery. 2021;**95**:106148

[17] Poget M, Chautems R, Kohler R, Diana M, Saadi A. Impact of the COVID-19 pandemic on the severity and management of acute appendicitis. Frontiers in Surgery. 2022;**9**:981885-981885

[18] Azadbakht M, Azadbakht S, Daniali S, Dehghani M. Comparison of the prevalence of perforated appendicitis during and before COVID19 pandemic. Annals of Medicine and Surgery. 2012;**2022**(82):104785-104785

[19] Tsou H, Huang S, Tsai C, Cheng S, Chu T. Outcomes of laparoscopic appendectomy during the level 3 alert of the coronavirus disease Pandemic in Taiwan: Experience in a referral center. Formosan Journal of Surgery. 2019;**2022**:134-139

[20] Nikolovski A, Ulusoy C, Dervishov K, Otljanski A. Acute appendicitis: Covid-19 pandemic did not change presentation and treatment. Annali Italiani di Chirurgia. 2022;**92**:369-373

[21] Bickel A, Ganam S, Shakra IA, et al. Delayed diagnosis and subsequently increased severity of acute appendicitis (compatible with clinical-pathologic grounds) during the COVID-19 pandemic: An observational case-control study. BMC Gastroenterology. 2022;**22**(1):NA-NA

[22] Herrera JJ, Arrechea R, Mihura M, Bregante M, Medina JP, Pirchi DE. Impact of the COVID-19 pandemic and restrictive measures on acute appendicitis: Do not let your guard down. Journal of Minimal Access Surgery. 2022;**18**(4):539-544

[23] Passoni S, Giuliani M, Arigoni M. Increased incidence of complicated acute appendicitis after the first COVID-19 pandemic peak: Have patients a different attitude towards COVID-hospitals? British Journal of Surgery. 2021;**108**(Suppl. 4):znab202. 046

[24] Turhan N, Arıcan ÇD. The effects of COVID-19 pandemic on patients with acute appendicitis. Turkish Journal of Trauma & Emergency Surgery. 2022;**28**(6):756

[25] Pellicciaro M, Vanni G, Grande S, et al. Acute appendicitis during coronavirus disease 2019 (COVID-19): Increasing incidence of complicate appendicitis, severity and length of hospitalization. In vivo. 2022;**36**(3):1325-1332

[26] An S, Kim H, Jang S, Kim K. The impact of the coronavirus disease-19 pandemic on the clinical characteristics and treatment of adult patients with acute appendicitis. Frontiers in Surgery. 2022;**9**:878534-878534

[27] Chang Y, Chen L. Did the severity of appendicitis increase during the COVID-19 pandemic? PLoS One. 2022;**17**(2):e0263814-e0263e14

[28] Tamirian R, Klein M, Chui P, et al. Acute appendicitis during the COVID-19 pandemic: A multicenter, retrospective analysis from the US epicenter. The American Surgeon. 2023;**89**(6):2554-2562

[29] Scheijmans J, Borgstein A, Puylaert C, et al. Impact of the COVID-19 pandemic on incidence and severity of acute appendicitis: A comparison between 2019 and 2020. BMC Emergency Medicine. 2021;**21**(1):61-61

[30] Frankcombe D, Gauri N, Satchithanandha V, et al. Management of

acute appendicitis during the COVID-19 pandemic: A retrospective cohort study. BMC Surgery. 2022;**22**(1):393-393

[31] Al-Abid M, Petrucci R, Preda TC, Lord SJ, Lord RV. Reduced number of admissions with acute appendicitis but not severe acute appendicitis at two Sydney hospitals during the first COVID-19 lockdown period. ANZ Journal of Surgery. 2022;**92**(7-8):1737-1741

[32] Drysdale HR, Ooi S, Team R, Nagra S, Watters DA, Guest GD. Clinical activity and outcomes during Geelong's general surgery response to the coronavirus disease 2019 pandemic. ANZ Journal of Surgery. 2020;**90**:1573-1579

[33] Australian Consortium for Classification Development. The international statistical classification of diseases and related health problems, tenth revision, Australian modification (ICD-10-AM/ACHI/ACS). First Edition to Eleventh Edition [PDF on internet]. 2019. Available from: https://www.ihacpa.gov.au/sites/default/files/2022-08/icd-10-am_chronicle_-_eleventh_edition.pdf [Accessed: 23 April, 2023]

[34] SNOMED-CT AU. International Health Terminology Standards Developmemnt Organisation. 2023. Available from: https://ontoserver.csiro.au/shrimp/?concept=138875005&valueset=http%3A%2F%2Fsnomed.info%2Fsct%3Ffhir_vs [Accessed: 20 Februrary, 2023]

[35] The Jamovi Project Jamovi. (Version 2.3) [Computer Software]. 2022. Available from: https://www.jamovi.org

[36] AlHarmi RAR, Almahari SA, AlAradi J, Alqaseer A, AlJirdabi NS, Ahmed FA. Seasonal variation in cases of acute appendicitis. Surgery Research and Practice. 2021;**2021**:8811898

[37] Orthopoulos G, Santone E, Izzo F, et al. Increasing incidence of complicated appendicitis during COVID-19 pandemic. The American Journal of Surgery. 2021;**221**(5):1056-1060

[38] Weinandt M, Godiris-Petit G, Menegaux F, Chereau N, Lupinacci RM. Appendicitis is a severe disease in elderly patients: A twenty-year audit. JSLS: Journal of the Society of Laparoendoscopic Surgeons. 2020;**24**(3):e2020.00046

[39] Lapsa S, Ozolins A, Strumfa I, Gardovskis J. Acute appendicitis in the elderly: A literature review on an increasingly frequent surgical problem. Geriatrics (Basel, Switzerland). 2021;**6**(3):93-93

[40] Willms AG, Oldhafer KJ, Conze S, et al. Appendicitis during the COVID-19 lockdown: Results of a multicenter analysis in Germany. Langenbeck's Archives of Surgery. 2021;**406**(2):367-375

[41] Oxenham M, Jull P, Karunaratne D, Laskar N, Harshen R. 720 outcomes of conservative Management of Acute Appendicitis during the COVID-19 pandemic. British Journal of Surgery. 2021;**108**(Suppl. 2):znab134. 078

[42] Iftikhar M, Shah S, Shah I, Shah J, Faisal M. Outcomes of conservative Management of Acute Appendicitis during COVID-19 pandemic. Journal of the College of Physicians and Surgeons–Pakistan: JCPSP. 2021;**31**(1):S50-S54

[43] Emile SH, Hamid HK, Khan SM, Davis GN. Rate of application and outcome of non-operative management of acute appendicitis in the setting of COVID-19: Systematic review and meta-analysis. Journal of Gastrointestinal Surgery. 2021;**25**(7):1905-1915

[44] Javanmard-Emamghissi H, Boyd-Carson H, Hollyman M, et al. The management of adult appendicitis during the COVID-19 pandemic: An interim analysis of a UK cohort study. Techniques in Coloproctology. 2021;**25**(4):401-411

[45] Burgard M, Cherbanyk F, Nassiopoulos K, Malekzadeh S, Pugin F, Egger B. An effect of the COVID-19 pandemic: Significantly more complicated appendicitis due to delayed presentation of patients. PLoS One. 2021;**16**(5):e0249171

[46] Baral S, Chhetri RK, Thapa N. Comparison of acute appendicitis before and within lockdown period in COVID-19 era: A retrospective study from rural Nepal. PLoS One. 2021;**16**(1):e0245137

Chapter 2

Diagnosis and Management of Acute Appendicitis

Mekki Hassan, Zafir Babiker and Mohamed Alfatih Hamza

Abstract

Acute appendicitis remains the most common indication for urgent abdominal surgery, with significant variations in presentation across different patient populations. This chapter provides a comprehensive overview of acute appendicitis's epidemiology, anatomy, pathogenesis, and clinical features, emphasising its diagnostic challenges, particularly in paediatric, elderly, and pregnant patients. Imaging modalities—including ultrasound, computed tomography (CT), and magnetic resonance imaging (MRI)—are explored in guiding diagnosis and management. Treatment approaches are reviewed, highlighting both operative (laparoscopic and open appendectomy) and non-operative management strategies, along with criteria for patient selection. The discussion extends to special considerations such as gangrenous appendicitis, appendiceal mass, and the role of interval appendectomy. Additionally, screening for malignancy in older patients is addressed, reinforcing the importance of individualised management. Advances in diagnostic tools and treatment protocols continue to refine clinical decision-making, reducing morbidity and improving patient outcomes.

Keywords: nonoperative management (NOM), operative management, antibiotics, appendectomy, laparoscopic surgery, open appendectomy, imaging modalities, ultrasound (US), computed tomography (CT), magnetic resonance imaging (MRI), complicated appendicitis, uncomplicated appendicitis, recurrence rate, timing of surgery, special populations (children, pregnant women, elderly)

1. Introduction

Acute appendicitis is an indication for urgent abdominal surgery, and it occurs at a rate of 5.7 to 50 cases per 100,000 individuals annually. The condition is more prevalent in the second and third decades of life. Males are slightly more likely to be affected, with a 1.5:1 male-to-female ratio [1].

Diagnosing acute appendicitis is most challenging at the extremes of age—difficult in young children due to the lack of a clear history and in the elderly because of a broad range of possible diagnoses and subtle or absent physical signs.

The mortality risk for acute non-gangrenous appendicitis is below 0.1%, but this risk increases to 0.6% in cases of gangrenous appendicitis. In contrast, perforated appendicitis has a significantly higher mortality rate of approximately 5% [2].

IntechOpen

2. Anatomy

The appendix is situated at the base of the cecum, near the ileocecal valve, where the taenia coli converge.

The blood supply of the appendix is from the appendiceal artery, which is a terminal branch of the ileocolic artery.

The location of the appendix can vary with positions including retrocecal, subcecal, retroileal, pre-ileal and pelvic.

These variations in location can influence the presentation of the condition because the site of pain and clinical exam findings are often indicative of the appendix's anatomical location.

3. Pathogenesis

Acute appendicitis usually begins with appendiceal lumen obstruction with inflammation of the appendiceal wall and then progresses to congestion. This rise in pressure results in thrombosis and occlusion of the small vessels within the appendiceal wall and localised ischemia, perforation, and may ultimately lead to the formation of a contained abscess or generalised peritonitis.

As the appendix becomes engorged, visceral afferent nerve fibres are stimulated, causing poorly localised central or periumbilical abdominal pain. Later in the disease course, as the inflammation spreads to the adjacent parietal peritoneum, pain becomes more well-localised.

In cases of gangrenous or perforated appendicitis, the most involved organisms include *Escherichia coli*, *Bacteroides fragilis*, and *Pseudomonas* species [3].

4. Causes

Luminal obstruction is commonly caused by fecaliths (hard faecal matter and inorganic salts), found in approximately 1/3 of acute appendicitis cases. Other causes of luminal obstruction include benign or malignant tumours of the appendix and cecum and lymphoid hyperplasia within the appendiceal wall.

Infectious causes include bacterial infections such as *Campylobacter*, *Brucella*, and *Salmonella*; parasitic infestations, including *Entamoeba histolytica*, *Schistosoma mansoni*, and *Enterobius vermicularis*.

4.1 Clinical features

Abdominal pain is the most common symptom of acute appendicitis, reported in nearly all confirmed cases. The typical presentation of acute appendicitis includes a combination of the following classic symptoms of right iliac fossa pain. Initially, periumbilical pain migrates to the RIF in 4–24 hours as the inflammation progresses. Although migratory pain is considered a hallmark symptom, it occurs in only 50–60% of patients with acute appendicitis with associate anorexia, nausea, vomiting and low-grade fever.

The symptoms can vary depending on the anatomical location of the appendix. For instance, an inflamed anterior appendix causes localised pain in RIF, while a retrocecal appendix may result in a more diffuse, dull abdominal pain [4]. When the tip of the appendix is in the pelvis, the pain can be atypical, with tenderness below McBurney's point. In these cases, patients may also experience urinary frequency, dysuria, or rectal symptoms such as tenesmus and diarrhoea.

In female patients, a detailed gynaecological history is essential, including information about menstrual cycles, vaginal discharge, or any history of conditions such as endometriosis.

The early physical signs of appendicitis can be mild in the initial stages, with minimal clinical findings. Signs include tachycardia, low-grade fever, and localised tenderness at the right iliac fossa (McBurney's point tenderness). Sensitivity ranges from 50% to 94% and specificity from 75% to 86% [5]: as the inflammation progresses, the parietal peritoneum becomes involved.

Other physical signs commonly associated with appendicitis (although their diagnostic value should be interpreted with caution, as these findings predate the use of imaging and vary widely in sensitivity and specificity): Psoas sign: Pain in the right lower quadrant with passive right hip extension, typically associated with a retrocecal appendix. Sensitivity is 13–42%, and specificity is 79–97% [5]. Obturator sign: Pain in the right lower quadrant when the right hip is flexed and internally rotated, indicating a pelvic appendix. Sensitivity is 8%, but specificity is 94% [5]. A rectal examination does not add diagnostic value in appendicitis.

Pelvic examination in women may reveal tenderness in the right adnexal region, making it difficult to distinguish between gynaecological and appendiceal causes of pain.

The Jerusalem guidelines, established by the World Society of Emergency Surgery (WSES), recommend utilising scoring systems such as the Alvarado score, the Adult Appendicitis Score (AAS), and the Appendicitis Inflammatory Response (AIR) to aid in the clinical diagnosis of acute appendicitis (AA) [6]. These scoring systems provide and guide an approach to diagnosing appendicitis, reducing admissions, optimising the utility of diagnostic imaging, and preventing negative surgical explorations, but none of these scoring systems are widely accepted for use [7, 8].

4.2 Differential diagnosis

Differentials to consider includes lymphadenitis, urinary tract infection/right-sided ureteric stones, distal ileum inflammatory bowel disease, terminal ileitis, right-sided colitis, diverticulitis [9] and gynaecological diseases (mainly ectopic pregnancy, ovarian cyst/torsion or haemorrhage, acute salpingitis, Mittelschmerz (mid-cycle) pain and pelvic inflammatory disease).

One of the most difficult differential diagnoses of acute appendicitis is acute Crohn's disease. A history of Crohn's disease may prevent unnecessary surgical procedures in the setting of acute abdominal pain as Crohn's disease can initially present like acute appendicitis. During the operation, inflammation of ileal loops could point towards Crohn's disease [10].

A good history and examination are necessary to manage the differential diagnosis such as recent viral infection causing mesenteric adenitis. Acute bacterial ileitis may be due to infections with Yersinia or Campylobacter. Also, severe cervical motion tenderness during the bimanual pelvic examination may indicate pelvic inflammatory disease [10].

5. Investigations

5.1 Lab investigations

Normal white cell count (WCC) cannot exclude AA, especially in the early stage, as WCC increases as AA progresses. A mild elevation in white cell count (WCC) above 10,000 cells/μL is common, with leucocytosis and neutrophilia. The sensitivity and specificity of elevated WBC levels for diagnosing appendicitis are 80% and 55%, respectively. Urinalysis is essential, particularly in women. Although pus cells and microscopic haematuria can occur in appendicitis, their absence may be useful in excluding significant urinary tract disease. Urinary or serum B-HCG test should be performed to exclude.

5.2 Imaging of appendicitis

Acute appendicitis is one of the most prevalent causes of acute abdominal pain, necessitating rapid surgical operation. If ignored and left untreated, appendicitis can cause serious complications such as appendix perforation, abscess formation, and peritonitis, all of which dramatically increase patient morbidity and mortality. As a result, a timely and precise diagnosis is critical to avoiding these severe results. Imaging is critical in detecting appendicitis, especially in cases where symptoms are atypical or unclear. This is especially critical in special populations, including children, the elderly, and pregnant women, who may exhibit atypical symptoms or face increased risks from delayed diagnosis.

When diagnosing appendicitis, the following primary imaging modalities are typically used: Ultrasound (US), computed tomography (CT), magnetic resonance imaging (MRI) and other imaging techniques (i.e. plain radiography and nuclear medicine).

5.3 Ultrasound

Graded compression ultrasound uses gentle pressure to move gas-filled intestinal loops, improving the appendix's visibility. An inflamed appendix is a non-compressible tubular construction with a blind end located in the lower right quadrant > 6 mm in outer diameter. In cross-section, the target sign and the wall thicken (>2 mm). Enhanced vascularity was observed using colour Doppler imaging [11]. Appendicolith (fecalith) may be present. Inflammation may also be indicated by peri-appendiceal fluid collection in the form of unified echo texture in echogenic areas on ultrasonography [12], or echogenic mesenteric fat. The advantages include No ionising radiation exposure, which makes it safe for use in pregnant women and children. Dynamic assessment that can link areas of maximal tenderness with imaging findings in real time [13, 14]. However, the limitations are that the device's sensitivity and specificity vary depending on the operator; individuals with high body mass index or significant intestinal gas may have limited visibility. Studies have shown that ultrasound can diagnose appendicitis in both adults and children, with sensitivities ranging from 71% to 94% and specificities from 81% to 98% [15, 16].

5.4 Computed tomography (CT)

Intravenous contrast-enhanced CT enhances the visual quality of the surrounding structures and the appendix. Also, low-dose CT preserves diagnostic accuracy while exposing patients to less radiation. On the other hand, oral and rectal contrast is less frequently utilised because it takes longer to prepare and causes discomfort to the patient.

The diagnostic criteria include appendix diameter (>6 mm), thickening of the appendix wall, and fat stranding around the appendix, which suggests inflammation and appendicolith presence [17]. Computed tomography also detects complications such as phlegmon/abscess.

Enhancing walls and fluid accumulation, or perforation (free gas). The advantages include >95% sensitivity and specificity, thorough examination of the pelvis and abdomen that permits the discovery of alternate diagnoses, and quick acquisition speed. However, the limitations are exposure to ionising radiation, possible contrast reactions, and, because of radiation risks, use is restricted in children and pregnant women. CT imaging has been shown to reduce negative appendectomy rates and improve diagnostic accuracy in adults with suspected appendicitis [18, 19].

5.5 Magnetic resonance imaging

MRI sequences—T2-weighted imaging demonstrates structures that are filled with fluid without the use of contrast chemicals. Enhance identification of inflammation in fat planes with fat-suppressed sequences. In addition, diffusion-weighted imaging (DWI) locates regions of limited diffusion linked to inflammation.

Wall thickening, peri-appendiceal inflammation, and an enlarged appendix are like CT findings, but superior soft-tissue contrast enables in-depth visualisation. Also, it is non-radioactive; hence, it is safe to use during pregnancy, especially in the second and third trimesters. MRI is expensive and has restricted availability, extended periods for examinations, and sensitivity to movements from the patient, which may cause an image's quality degradation or movement artefacts.

MRI has been shown to have a high sensitivity and specificity for the diagnosis of appendicitis; it is particularly helpful in situations where ultrasound results are unclear and radiation exposure is a concern [20, 21].

5.6 Other imaging methods

5.6.1 Plain radiography

It has a limited role in diagnosing appendicitis and may exhibit indirect signs such as fecaliths, localised ileus, or elevated air-fluid levels. Low diagnostic yield implies that it is not usually suggested [22].

5.6.2 Nuclear medicine

Radionuclide imaging employs leukocytes that have been radiolabelled to identify inflammation. It is rarely utilised because of time constraints and the availability of imaging technologies that are more effective [23].

5.7 Special populations

5.7.1 Children

Ultrasound is the primary imaging modality for detecting appendicitis. It is non-invasive, free of radiation, and produces real-time findings, which is very useful in paediatric treatment. It enables viewing of the appendix and associated tissues, which aids in the rapid confirmation or exclusion of appendicitis; however, in many cases, the appendix is not readily visible, especially in younger children or those with a higher body mass index (BMI). In addition, Ultrasound sensitivity can be diminished in children who have trouble participating throughout the process since movement can distort pictures and impair diagnostic accuracy. Furthermore, if there is a lot of intestinal gas or an unusual appendix position, ultrasonography may not produce accurate data. Ultrasound is a highly successful diagnostic technique for paediatric appendicitis, with 88% sensitivity and 94% specificity. This implies that it correctly detects a lot of cases of appendicitis and reliably rules it out in healthy children [15].

CT is used cautiously, especially in older children or when other diagnostic methods are inconclusive. While it provides a more definitive diagnosis, its use is limited due to radiation exposure; therefore, it is used with caution.

MRI is a highly accurate and radiation-free option that can be applied when ultrasound and CT are ambiguous or when avoiding radiation is crucial, such as in young children or individuals with recurrent appendicitis.

5.7.2 Pregnant women

Ultrasound is the first line of imaging; second-line imaging is MRI without gadolinium contrast agents. CT is only used in pregnant women when an MRI is unavailable or unclear because it poses a foetal radiation exposure risk. It is a last choice after careful discussion with the patient, obstetrician and radiologist, intended for situations in which a correct diagnosis is critical to avoiding significant complications. If ultrasonography is nondiagnostic, MRI is safe to use during pregnancy and offers a precise diagnosis [20, 21].

5.7.3 Elderly

CT is recommended for elderly patients due to a higher risk of atypical presentations and other differentials such as diverticulitis and colonic cancer. It helps to confirm the diagnosis and rule out other possible sources of symptoms. When treating elderly individuals who may have appendicitis, CT imaging enhances diagnostic precision and management by providing a clear view of the appendix and surrounding structures; this enhanced accuracy allows for better decision-making regarding treatment [12].

5.8 Role of imaging in management

Diagnosis confirmation: Imaging plays an important role in management by accurately diagnosing appendicitis and minimising unnecessary surgeries such as negative appendectomies. It distinguishes appendicitis from other illnesses with similar symptoms.

Treatment planning: Imaging aids in planning treatment by detecting problems such as abscesses or perforations and exposing anatomical differences. This ensures that surgical and non-surgical procedures are adjusted for better results.

Nonoperative management: Antibiotics may be taken into consideration in certain cases of uncomplicated appendicitis; hence, imaging verifies that there is no abscess, perforation, or fecalith.

Follow up imaging facilitates evaluation of the response of patients receiving conservative treatment, such as antibiotic medication, and determining the need for surgical intervention. Specifically, imaging determines whether problems such as abscess formation, perforation, or increasing inflammation have developed, indicating that nonoperative treatment is no longer recommended. Imaging allows for quick and informed judgements, balancing the risks and advantages of nonoperative therapy versus surgical intervention.

Imaging-guided management techniques have decreased healthcare expenses and improved patient outcomes [24, 25].

5.9 Conclusion

To summarise, imaging modalities such as ultrasound, CT, MRI, and others are critical in the diagnosis and treatment of appendicitis. They help medical professionals make accurate diagnoses, plan appropriate treatment, and track progress, resulting in better patient outcomes and fewer wasteful operations.

6. Management of acute appendicitis

Management involves a combination of clinical evaluation, imaging, and tailored treatment approaches, depending on the severity and individual patient factors. The two primary strategies are nonoperative management (NOM) with antibiotics for selected uncomplicated cases and surgical intervention through appendectomy.

6.1 Nonoperative management

6.1.1 In adults

Adults who present with acute appendicitis can be managed non-operatively with antibiotics; careful selection criteria and discussion with the patient are needed prior to starting this treatment strategy. Selection criteria are CRP < 60 g/L, WBC < 12 × 109/L, and age < 60 years [26], duration of symptoms <24 hours, Alvarado score < 4. On the other hand, gangrenous appendix, large abscess, peritonitis, and pregnancy are contraindications according to the 2020 update of the WSES Jerusalem guidelines [27], together with the presence of a fecolith [28].

NOM carries a 1-year recurrence rate of 27.3%, of which the complicated acute appendicitis rate is 10% [29].

The duration of antibiotic therapy is 3–7 days; local hospital antimicrobial guidance will be a good reference for antibiotic choice and route.

Benefits and risks [30] of NOM include a return to work: 1.78 days shorter, and the need for a new course of antibiotics: 9 fewer per 1000, but there are risks of readmission: 201 more per 1000, post-treatment abscess: 9 more per 1000, need for IR drainage: 14 more per 1000 and conversion to operative management or reoperation: 91 more per 1000.

Overall, careful discussion with patients/guardians is crucial in the decision-making process of NOM of acute appendicitis.

6.1.2 In paediatrics

Paediatric acute appendicitis can also be treated as NOM with careful selection as well.

Selection criteria are uncomplicated AA without an appendicolith [31]. Appendectomy avoidance rate is 62–81% after 1-year follow-up [32]. Antibiotic therapy duration is 3–7 days; local hospital antimicrobial policy will be a good reference for antibiotics route and choice.

Benefits and risks [30] of NOM in paediatrics include the return to school: 2 days shorter, ICU admission: 39 fewer per 1000. Post-treatment abscess: 18 fewer per 1000 and need for IR drainage: 8 fewer per 1000. However, the length of stay is 1.4 days longer, and the readmission rate is 220 more per 1000.

Overall, careful discussion with patients/guardians is crucial in the decision-making process of NOM of acute appendicitis.

6.2 Operative treatment of acute appendicitis

6.2.1 Timing of surgery

Data from the American College of Surgeons NSQIP demonstrated no increase in complications if appendectomy for AA was performed on hospital day 1 or 2; however, appendectomies performed on hospital day 3 had worse outcomes, increased 30-day mortality (0.6%), and all major postoperative complications (8%) in comparison with operations taking place on hospital day 1 (0.1%; 3.4%) or 2 (0.1%; 3.6%). Risk is higher in patients with increased ASA.

The American Paediatric Surgical Association Outcomes recommendations: Appendectomy performed within the first 24 hours from presentation is not associated with an increased risk of perforation or adverse outcomes.

6.2.2 Laparoscopic versus open appendectomy

Laparoscopic appendectomy offers significant advantages over open appendectomy in terms of less pain, lower incidence of surgical site infection, decreased length of hospital stay, earlier return to work, overall costs, and better quality of life scores [27].

6.2.3 Laparoscopic appendicectomy

Preoperative adequate resuscitation, IV antibiotics, analgesia, VTE prophylaxis, consent, and anaesthetic review (WHO checklist).

Incision can be either standard, supra/infraumbilical open Hasson Technique to insert a camera port and x2 additional ports—two 5 mm or 10 and 5 mm according to operator preference, generally positioned in the left iliac fossa and suprapubic area; position may vary according to operator preference. Single-incision laparoscopic appendectomy (SILA); is another effective way to perform appendectomy; however, it has a higher incidence of SSI compared with three-port LA and requires a longer operative time [33].

Laparoscopy: Conduct quick diagnostic laparoscopy; a gentle head-down and right-side-up position will help in displaying the pelvis and easy identification of the appendix.

Intraoperative appendicitis grading: Commonly used systems are WSES grading: grade 0 (normal), grade 1 (inflamed), grade 2 (necrosis), grade 3 (inflammatory tumour), and grade 4 (peritonitis), and AAST grading: ranging from grade 1 (mild) to grade V (severe).

Intraoperatively normal appendix: The European Association of Endoscopic Surgery (EAES) 2016 guidelines recommended performing an appendectomy in the case of a normal-appearing appendix during surgery for suspected AA in the absence of other pathology. Lavage and suction or suction alone (no difference) [30].

Control of mesoappendix: Thin mesoappendix can be controlled using endoclip, endoloop, and electrocoagulation. However, thick/gangrenous mesoappendix: Harmonic Scalpel, or *LigaSure* (higher cost).

Stump Closure: The infectious complication rate is not influenced by the type of appendicular stump closure [34]; techniques used in uncomplicated appendicitis are endoloop, ligation, and clips, including polymeric clips. In complicated appendicitis, an endostapler can be used.

Drains associated with increased hospital stay and did not reduce postoperative intraabdominal abscess [35].

6.2.4 Open appendectomy

Incision: A right lower quadrant transverse incision (McBurney's) is preferred for its direct access and cosmetic considerations. Alternatively, a right lower quadrant Lanz incision or midline incision may be used in certain cases. Dissection and Exposure, Layer-by-Layer Dissection; Skin and Subcutaneous Tissue: Incise the skin and subcutaneous tissues, separate the external oblique, internal oblique, and transversus abdominis muscles along their natural lines (blunt dissection), then incise the fascia and peritoneum to enter the abdominal cavity.

Handling adhesions: If the appendix is adherent to surrounding structures (common in complicated appendicitis), carefully dissect adhesions using sharp and blunt dissection techniques to avoid injury to adjacent organs. Locate the appendix; identify the cecum, typically found in the right lower quadrant. The appendix appears as a narrow, finger-like projection from the cecum at the end of the taenia coli. Gently mobilise the cecum if necessary to expose the base of the appendix and carefully isolate the appendix from the cecum.

Place ligatures (e.g. absorbable sutures) around the base of the appendix and mesoappendix to control blood supply and prevent leakage. Divide the mesoappendix (the connective tissue attaching the appendix to the ileum and containing blood vessels) using electrocautery or scissors. Inspect the abdominal cavity for any signs of perforation, abscess, or contamination. Irrigate the area with saline if necessary and ensure all bleeding sources are controlled.

Layered closure: Close the peritoneal layer if disrupted and approximate and suture the fascia with non-absorbable or slowly absorbable sutures. Close the subcutaneous layer using absorbable sutures or staples then close the skin with sutures, staples, or adhesive strips, depending on surgeon preference and patient factors.

6.2.5 Postoperative antibiotics

In complicated appendicitis, a course of 3–5 days according to STOP IT RCT [36]. However, in uncomplicated appendicitis it is not recommended and only a single dose from 0 to 60 minutes prior to skin incision (WSES guidelines).

In adults, there is emerging evidence that oral antibiotics may be as effective as IV antibiotics [37]; however, the current evidence supports IV antibiotics for 48 hours, then an oral switch when clinically justifiable [38]. In children, an early oral switch is as soon as the patient is ready for discharge [39].

6.3 Gangrenous appendicitis

It occurs in 17% of cases of acute appendicitis and is associated with increased rates of complications such as intraabdominal abscesses and appendiceal perforation if surgical management is delayed. Intraluminal air, along with other radiological and clinical features, serves as an indicator of gangrenous appendicitis [40]. Preoperative high Total Bilirubin >1 mg/dL could be useful to diagnose gangrenous appendicitis [41]. In line with WSES guidelines 2020 patients with suspected gangrenous appendicitis should be treated with appendicectomy.

6.4 Appendix mass/abscess

An appendiceal mass usually comprises the inflamed appendix, surrounding omentum, and sometimes adjacent structures forming a localised inflammatory process.

An appendiceal abscess typically forms when an inflamed appendix perforates, leading to localised collection of pus surrounded by inflamed tissues.

Nonoperative treatment with antibiotics is recommended as first-line treatment, succeeding in over 90% of patients with an overall risk of recurrence of 7.4% and only 19.7% of cases of abscess requiring percutaneous drainage [42], also associated with less wound infection, abdominal/pelvic abscess, ileus, and reoperation rate [43]. Another piece of evidence suggests that recurrence after non-surgical treatment is as high as 12% [44]. IR drainage is recommended if the abscess is large (typically >3–4 cm) or if there is no significant clinical improvement with antibiotic therapy alone.

Surgical treatment (laparoscopic or open) is indicated in the presence of generalised peritonitis, hemodynamic instability or if the patient does not respond to initial antibiotic therapy and is not IR-drainable.

In the presence of advanced lap expertise, this may be considered as a first-line surgical strategy [45].

6.5 Interval appendectomy

The surgical morbidity rate of appendectomy is 12.4% [42]. Therefore, interval appendectomy is considered in specific clinical scenarios where immediate surgery may carry higher risks or when nonoperative management has been initially successful, typically performed after 6–8 weeks.

According to WSES Jerusalem guidelines, 2020 indicated only patients with recurrent symptoms.

7. Screening for cancer

The risk of malignancy is about 3% in patients above the age of 40 [46].

Colonic screening with colonoscopy and interval full-dose contrast-enhanced CT scan for patients with appendicitis treated non-operatively if ≥40 years old is recommended by WSES Jerusalem guidelines 2020.

8. Conclusion

Nonoperative management (NOM) provides an alternative for selected uncomplicated cases, offering reduced recovery times but with higher recurrence risks. Operative management through laparoscopic or open appendectomy remains the gold standard, particularly for complicated cases or those with recurrent symptoms.

Tailoring treatment to specific populations, such as children, pregnant women, and the elderly, ensures optimal outcomes by balancing diagnostic accuracy with patient safety. Early diagnosis, guided by clinical assessment and imaging combined with timely intervention, is pivotal in minimising complications and improving overall patient outcomes.

Conflict of interest

No.

Abbreviations

NOM	nonoperative management
US	ultrasound
CT	computed tomography
MRI	magnetic resonance imaging
CRP	C-reactive protein
WBC	white blood cell
SSI	surgical site infection
SILA	single-incision laparoscopic appendectomy
IR	interventional radiology
VTE	venous thromboembolism

Author details

Mekki Hassan[1*], Zafir Babiker[2] and Mohamed Alfatih Hamza[3]

1 Hull University Teaching Hospitals Trust, Northern Care Alliance NHS, Hull, England

2 Aneurin Bevan University Health Board, Newport, United Kingdom

3 Mersey and West Lancashire NHS Trust, Whiston and St Helens Hospital, England

*Address all correspondence to: mekkihasssan@yahoo.com

IntechOpen

© 2025 The Author(s). Licensee IntechOpen. This chapter is distributed under the terms of the Creative Commons Attribution License (http://creativecommons.org/licenses/by/4.0), which permits unrestricted use, distribution, and reproduction in any medium, provided the original work is properly cited.

References

[1] Cervellin G, Mora R, Ticinesi A, et al. Epidemiology and outcomes of acute abdominal pain in a large urban emergency department: Retrospective analysis of 5,340 cases. Annals of Translational Medicine. 2016;**4**:362

[2] Livingston EH, Woodward WA, Sarosi GA, et al. Disconnect between incidence of nonperforated and perforated appendicitis: Implications for pathophysiology and management. Annals of Surgery. 2007;**245**:886-892

[3] Bennion RS, Baron EJ, Thompson JE Jr, et al. The bacteriology of gangrenous and perforated appendicitis—Revisited. Annals of Surgery. 1990;**211**:165

[4] Guidry SP, Poole GV. The anatomy of appendicitis. The American Surgeon. 1994;**60**:68

[5] Golledge J, Toms AP, Franklin IJ, et al. Assessment of peritonism in appendicitis. Annals of the Royal College of Surgeons of England. 1996;**78**:11

[6] Di Saverio S, Podda M, De Simone B, Ceresoli M, Augustin G, Gori A, et al. Diagnosis and treatment of acute appendicitis: 2020 update of the WSES Jerusalem guidelines. World Journal of Emergency Surgery. 2020;(15):1-42

[7] Andersson M, Andersson RE. The appendicitis inflammatory response score: A tool for the diagnosis of acute appendicitis that outperforms the Alvarado score. World Journal of Surgery. 2008;**32**:1843-1849

[8] Alvarado A. A practical score for the early diagnosis of acute appendicitis. Annals of Emergency Medicine. 1986;**15**:557-564

[9] Humes DJ, Simpson J. Acute appendicitis. BMJ. 2006;**333**(7567):530-534. DOI: 10.1136/bmj.38940.664363.AE

[10] Lotfollahzadeh, Saran, Richard A. Lopez, and Jeffrey G. Deppen. "Appendicitis." In StatPearls. Treasure Island (FL): StatPearls Publishing; 12 February 2024. Available from: Available from: https://www.ncbi.nlm.nih.gov/books/NBK493193/

[11] Watanabe K, Aizawa T. Ultrasound findings in acute appendicitis: A review. Journal of Medical Ultrasonics. 2020;**47**(1):1-8

[12] Fugazzola P, Ceresoli M, Agnoletti V, et al. The SIFIPAC/WSES/SICG/SIMEU guidelines for diagnosis and treatment of acute appendicitis in the elderly (2019 edition). World Journal of Emergency Surgery. 2020;**15**(1)

[13] Granata C et al. Let's talk about radiation dose and radiation protection in children. Pediatric Radiology. 2024;**55**(3):386-396. DOI: 10.1007/s00247-024-06009-0

[14] Tomà P et al. Protecting sensitive patient groups from imaging using ionizing radiation: Effects during pregnancy, in fetal life and childhood. La Radiologia Medica. 2019;**124**(8):736-744. DOI: 10.1007/s11547-019-01034-8

[15] Doria AS, Moineddin R, Kellenberger CJ, et al. US or CT for diagnosis of appendicitis in children and adults? A meta-analysis. Radiology. 2006;**241**(1):83-94

[16] Kaiser S, Frenckner B, Jorulf HK. Suspected appendicitis in children: US and CT—A prospective randomized study. Radiology. 2002;**223**(3):633-638

[17] Balthazar EJ, Megibow AJ. Imaging of appendicitis. Radiology. 2019;**292**(1):25-40

[18] Raman SS, Lu DS, Kadell BM. Accuracy of nonfocused helical CT for the diagnosis of acute appendicitis: A 5-year review. AJR. American Journal of Roentgenology. 2002;**178**(6):1319-1325

[19] Rao PM, Rhea JT, Novelline RA, et al. Helical CT technique for the diagnosis of appendicitis: Prospective evaluation of a focused appendix CT examination. Radiology. 1997;**202**(1):139-144

[20] Pedrosa I, Zeikus EA, Levine D, et al. MR imaging evaluation of acute appendicitis in pregnancy. Radiology. 2006;**238**(3):891-899

[21] Israel GM, Malguria N, McCarthy S, Copel J, Weinreb J. MRI vs. Ultrasound for Suspected Appendicitis During Pregnancy. Journal of Magnetic Resonance Imaging. 2008;**28**(2):428-433. DOI: 10.1002/jmri.21456

[22] Baker SR. Acute appendicitis: Plain radiographic considerations. Emergency Radiology. 1996;**3**(2):63-69. DOI: 10.1007/bf01507935

[23] Meibom SK, Benador-Shen IY, Mercier GA. 111Indium-labeled leukocyte imaging of infection and inflammation. In Nuclear Medicine and Immunology. Springer; 2021. pp. 125-152. DOI: 10.1007/978-3-030-81261-4_5

[24] Tierney MC. Patient Pathways & Better Outcomes: The Future of Radiology. HealthManagement.org, 2016. Available from: https://healthmanagement.org/c/imaging/whitepaper/patient-pathways-better-outcomes-the-future-of-radiology [Accessed April 11, 2025]

[25] Sorger JM. How to objectively evaluate the impact of image-guided surgery technologies. European Journal of Nuclear Medicine and Molecular Imaging. 2023;**51**(10):2869-2877. DOI: 10.1007/s00259-023-06504-w

[26] Hansson J, Körner U, Khorram-Manesh A, Solberg A, Lundholm K. Randomized clinical trial of antibiotic therapy versus appendicectomy as primary treatment of acute appendicitis in unselected patients. The British Journal of Surgery. 2009;**96**(5):473-481. DOI: 10.1002/bjs.6482

[27] Di Saverio S, Podda M, De Simone B, Ceresoli M, Augustin G, Gori A, et al. Diagnosis and treatment of acute appendicitis: 2020 update of the WSES Jerusalem guidelines. World Journal of Emergency Surgery. 2020;**15**:27

[28] Mällinen J, Vaarala S, Mäkinen M, Lietzén E, Grönroos J, Ohtonen P, et al. Appendicolith appendicitis is clinically complicated acute appendicitis—Is it histopathologically different from uncomplicated acute appendicitis. International Journal of Colorectal Disease. 2019;**34**(8):1393-1400. DOI: 10.1007/s00384-019-03332-z

[29] Salminen P, Paajanen H, Rautio T, Nordström P, Aarnio M, Rantanen T, et al. Antibiotic therapy vs appendectomy for treatment of uncomplicated acute appendicitis: The APPAC randomized clinical trial. JAMA. 2015;**313**(23):2340-2348. DOI: 10.1001/jama.2015.6154

[30] Kumar SS, Collings AT, Ryan Lamm MD, Haskins IN, Scholz S, Nepal P, et al. SAGES guideline for the diagnosis and treatment of appendicitis. Surgical Endoscopy. 2024;**38**(6):2974-2994. DOI: 10.1007/s00464-024-10813-y

[31] Huang L, Yin Y, Yang L, Wang C, Li Y, Zhou Z. Comparison of antibiotic

therapy and appendectomy for acute uncomplicated appendicitis in children: A meta-analysis. JAMA Pediatrics. 2017;**171**(5):426-434

[32] Gorter RR, Eker HH, Gorter-Stam MAW, Abis GSA, Acharya A, Ankersmit M, et al. Diagnosis and management of acute appendicitis. EAES consensus development conference 2015. Surgical Endoscopy. 2015;**11**:4668-4690

[33] Xue C, Lin B, Huang Z, Chen Z. Single-incision laparoscopic appendectomy versus conventional 3-port laparoscopic appendectomy for appendicitis: An updated meta-analysis of randomized controlled trials. Surgery Today. 2015;**45**(9):1179-1186

[34] Swank HA, van Rossem CC, van Geloven AW, in't Hof KH, Kazemier G, Meijerink WJHJ, et al. Endostapler or endoloops for securing the appendiceal stump in laparoscopic appendectomy: A retrospective cohort study. Surgical Endoscopy. 2014;**28**(2):576-583. DOI: 10.1007/s00464-013-3207-x

[35] Abu A, Mohamedahmed AY, Alamin A, Mohamed M, Osman M, Mohammed MJ, et al. Evaluation of drain insertion after appendicectomy for complicated appendicitis: A systematic review and meta-analysis. Cureus. 2022;**14**(11):e32018. DOI: 10.7759/cureus.32018

[36] Sawyer RG, Claridge JA, Nathens AB, Rotstein OD, Duane TM, Evans HL, et al. Trial of short-course antimicrobial therapy for intraabdominal infection. The New England Journal of Medicine. 2015;**372**(21):1996-2005. DOI: 10.1056/NEJMoa1411162

[37] Lipping E, Saar S, Reinsoo A, Bahhir A, Kirsimägi Ü, Lepner U, et al. Short postoperative intravenous versus oral antibacterial therapy in complicated acute appendicitis: A pilot noninferiority randomized trial. Annals of Surgery. 2024, 2024;**279**(2):191-195

[38] Sevinç F, Prins JM, Koopmans RP, Langendijk PN, Dankert J, Speelman P. Early change from intravenous to oral antibiotics: 'switch therapy'. Nederlands Tijdschrift voor Geneeskunde. 1999;**143**(47):2364-2369

[39] Arnold MR, Wormer BA, Kao AM, Klima DA, Colavita PD, Cosper GH, et al. Home intravenous versus oral antibiotics following appendectomy for perforated appendicitis in children: A randomized controlled trial. Pediatric Surgery International. 2018, 2018;**34**(12):1257-1268

[40] Ip C, Wang EH, Croft M, Lim W. Appendiceal intraluminal gas: A CT marker for gangrenous appendicitis. Radiology Research and Practice. 2021. Article ID 7191348. DOI: 10.1155/2021/7191348

[41] Naya I, Adachi K, Takeuchi K, Ariyama Y, Hosaka A, Imamura K, et al. Clinical predictors of gangrenous appendicitis: Elevated total bilirubin level and computed tomography scan findings. Acute Medicine & Surgery. 2021;**8**(1):e620. DOI: 10.1002/ams2.620

[42] Andersson RE, Petzold MG. Nonsurgical treatment of appendiceal abscess or phlegmon: A systematic review and meta-analysis. Annals of Surgery. 2007;**246**(5):741-748

[43] Federico C, Paola F, Massimo S, Enrico C, Maria GS, Gioacchino L, et al. Conservative treatment of acute appendicitis. Acta Bio-Medica. 2018;**89**(Suppl. 9):119-134

[44] Darwazeh G, Cunningham SC, Kowdley GC. A systematic review of

perforated appendicitis and phlegmon: Interval appendectomy or wait-and-see? The American Surgeon. 2016;**82**(1):11-15

[45] Mentula P, Sammalkorpi H, Leppäniemi A. Laparoscopic surgery or conservative treatment for appendiceal abscess in adults? A randomized controlled trial. Annals of Surgery. 2015;**262**(2):237-242

[46] Renteria O, Shahid Z, Huerta S. Outcomes of appendectomy in elderly veteran patients. Surgery. 2018;**164**(3):460-446

Chapter 3

Treatment of Acute Appendicitis

Summi Karn, Navin Kumar, Karamveer Singh and Somprakas Basu

Abstract

Treatment of appendicitis is continuously evolving. Appendectomy remains the standard for acute cases, whereas antibiotics are increasingly explored for uncomplicated appendicitis, showing comparable short-term outcomes. Around 25% eventually requires surgery within a year. Conservative antibiotic therapy, targeting aerobic and anaerobic bacteria, is viable for selected cases, particularly those without complicating factors. Complicated appendicitis warrants emergency appendectomy, laparoscopic or open. Appendicular lumps are often treated conservatively initially in both complicated and uncomplicated appendicitis, followed by interval appendectomy if risk factors persist. Debates persist over missed malignancies and long-term efficacy with conservative management, despite benefits like reduced pain and quicker recovery compared to surgery. Introduction of routine CT scans can increase success rate of conservative management by identifying underlying pathologies and risk factors for recurrences. Surgical removal remains dominant due to historically higher success rates and concerns over missing neoplasms. Nonetheless, antibiotics present a safe alternative for carefully selected patients.

Keywords: appendicitis, appendectomy, antibiotics therapy, conservative management, nonoperative management

1. Introduction

The management of appendicitis has undergone significant evolution over the years. Historically, acute appendicitis has been treated by an appendectomy, a surgical removal of the appendix. The first documented successful appendectomy was performed in 1735 by Claudius Amyand. Later, in 1880, Robert Lawson Tait was the first to make the diagnosis of appendicitis and performed the surgical removal of the appendix. In 1886, Reginald Heber Fitz contributed to the field by publishing a seminal study on appendicitis and coined the term "appendectomy" to describe the surgical procedure [1].

Appendectomy remains the standard for managing acute cases even today, particularly in cases with severe or complicated presentations. Nevertheless, contemporary understanding has differentiated appendicitis into two main categories: uncomplicated and complicated. Each category has distinct clinical trajectories, prognostic implications, and management strategies [2].

Recent research has increasingly explored the role of antibiotic therapy as a viable treatment modality for uncomplicated appendicitis. Advances in both diagnostic techniques and treatment options have expanded the range of management strategies, including the use of antibiotics alone in select cases. Studies conducted over the past two decades suggest that conservative management with antibiotics can yield comparable short-term outcomes to surgical intervention in select cases. This approach has gained traction, as many patients with uncomplicated appendicitis can achieve resolution of their symptoms without the need for an operative procedure. In such cases, appendectomy may be deemed unnecessary and potentially counterproductive.

Ultrasonography (USG) abdomen, being a non-invasive and radiation-free modality, offers a valuable modality in the diagnosis of acute appendicitis. However, its effectiveness is operator-dependent and may be limited in obese patients or those with retrocecal appendices. Nevertheless, USG remains the first investigation in any patient presenting with right lower abdominal pain. The integration of routine abdominal computed tomography (CT) scans has further refined the management approach by enhancing the identification of underlying pathologies and assessing risk factors for recurrence [1]. This diagnostic tool improves the accuracy of conservative treatment plans and helps tailor patient management strategies.

The choice between surgical intervention and conservative management is influenced by various factors, including the patient's overall health, the severity of symptoms, and the presence of complications such as abscess formation or perforation. Understanding the complexities of acute appendicitis and its management is crucial for optimizing patient outcomes and reducing the risk of complications. It includes recognizing the clinical presentation, utilizing appropriate diagnostic tools, and selecting the most effective treatment approach based on individual patient circumstances. The management strategies for the different presentations of appendicitis are discussed in detail within this section.

2. Uncomplicated appendicitis

Traditionally, appendectomy has been the standard of care even for uncomplicated appendicitis. However, in recent years, the management of acute appendicitis nonoperatively with antibiotics alone has emerged as a viable treatment option, particularly for uncomplicated cases. Conservative or nonoperative management primarily involves the use of antibiotics as an alternative to surgical intervention. This approach aims to resolve inflammation and infection without the need for surgical intervention, thus reducing the immediate risks and recovery time associated with surgery. Even though appendectomy is well-tolerated major surgical intervention but can lead to postoperative morbidity.

Antibiotic therapy can be effective and safe. Empiric antibiotic regimens are designed to target the polymicrobial flora commonly found in the appendiceal lumen. Current protocols usually involve a combination of broad-spectrum antibiotics. Despite the effectiveness and safety of this approach, a notable concern is the risk of recurrence. The APPAC RCT, for instance, reported a 39.1% recurrence rate within 5 years. Given that only about 20% of all participants present with complicated appendicitis, this shift in the treatment strategy for most patients with uncomplicated appendicitis can have wide reaching consequences [3].

The growing number of available broad-spectrum antibiotics has made antibiotic therapy increasingly attractive. Katie et al. conducted a meta-analysis and found that antibiotics are safe and effective as primary treatment. This analysis found a 52% reduction in risk of requiring an appendectomy, with one-year follow-up showing treatment efficacy in the antibiotic group and in the appendectomy group of 62.6 and 88.1%, respectively [4]. However, concerns persist regarding the incidence of recurrent appendicitis. The APPAC I trial found that 73% of patients with uncomplicated acute appendicitis treated with antibiotics did not require subsequent appendectomy even up to 1 year follow-up. Furthermore, complications were minimal among those who eventually needed surgery, suggesting that antibiotics can be considered a safer first-line treatment for CT-proven uncomplicated appendicitis over emergency surgery. Majority of the patients receiving intravenous antibiotics did not require subsequent appendectomy for recurrent appendicitis during one-year follow-up. However, the result of this trial could not demonstrate the noninferiority of antibiotic therapy as compared to appendectomy [3].

The "Comparison of Outcomes of Antibiotic Drugs and Appendectomy (CODA) trial" done in adults with appendicitis compared antibiotic therapy with appendectomy. It concluded that the antibiotic therapy is noninferior to appendectomy, with 29% of antibiotic group undergoing appendectomy at 90 days, of which 41% had an appendicolith and 25% did not. Another perspective is that over 70% participants on antibiotics avoided surgery. Compared to those who underwent appendicectomy, majority were treated as outpatients, and both caregiver and patient returned to their work earlier [5].

Although evidences show that primary antibiotic therapy for uncomplicated appendicitis is safe and efficient, this approach has not been widely accepted. Challenges include the impracticality of routine CT scans for all patients with right lower abdomen pain and the concerns that complications might arise from antibiotic therapy alone. Many centers have started considering antibiotics for 24–48 hours following admission, continuing them if clinical status improves, or performing an appendectomy if the patient worsens. Nonoperative approach may offer benefits like earlier recovery and reduced days away from work. Appendectomy is reserved for cases that do not respond to antibiotics or have recurrences. Conservative treatment is not without its challenges, requiring careful patient selection and follow-up to monitor for recurrence, and further management if needed. These patients must be thoroughly informed about potential disease progression, the possibility of recurrences, and the risk of undiagnosed neoplasms.

2.1 Acute catarrhal appendicitis

Acute appendicitis is commonly associated with polymicrobial infection. The most common organism isolated is *Escherichia coli*, followed by *Klebsiella pneumoniae*, *Streptococci*, *Enterococci* and *Pseudomonas aeruginosa* [6]. Given the safety and cost-effectiveness of nonoperative treatment for uncomplicated appendicitis, it is crucial to optimize the antibiotic therapy focusing on both antibiotic spectrum and the duration. The antibiotic regimen should adequately cover gram-negative and gram-positive bacteria, as well as anaerobes.

Currently, there is no standardized antibiotic protocol for the management of acute appendicitis. The guideline for the management of intra-abdominal infection was revised by the Surgical Infection Society (SIS) in 2017. According to these guidelines, source control is recommended if there is any intraperitoneal collection, which does not apply to uncomplicated appendicitis. For uncomplicated cases, antibiotic regimen which is effective against the typical gram-negative bacilli, gram-positive cocci, and obligate anaerobes is suggested. Recommended treatment for lower-risk patients includes cefepime or ceftriaxone, amoxicillin-clavulanate, and fluoroquinolones in combination with metronidazole. Single agent therapies such as ertapenem or moxifloxacin are also considered effective. For higher risk patients, piperacillin-tazobactam or meropenem is advised as a single agent, or cefepime with metronidazole, or aztreonam with vancomycin [7].

The APPAC II trial compared the efficacy, post-intervention complications, length of hospital stay, and treatment costs between two groups (oral antibiotic monotherapy versus a combination of intravenous and oral antibiotics). Moxifloxacin 400 mg daily was given for 7 days as an oral regimen. The intravenous plus oral regimen included 2 days of intravenous ertapenem sodium 1 g daily, followed by 5 days of oral levofloxacin 500 mg daily and metronidazole 500 mg three times daily. The trial concluded that moxifloxacin is a practical choice for oral monotherapy due to its inclusion in "current practice guidelines for community-acquired intra-abdominal infections" [8] and has broad spectrum coverage with proven efficacy against facultative gram-negative aerobes and anaerobes [9, 10]. Additionally, the once-daily administration of moxifloxacin was considered an advantage [11].

Majority of trials follow antibiotic guidelines for community-acquired intra-abdominal infections provided by Infectious Diseases Society of America (IDSA) and Surgical Infection Society (SIS) [8]. They recommend combination therapy of a second- or third-generation cephalosporin (such as cefmetazole, ceftriaxone, or cefotaxime), with metronidazole or tinidazole as initial parenteral antibiotic regimens. Monotherapy included Beta-lactams (such as amoxicillin-clavulanate and piperacillin-tazobactam) or carbapenem (such as ertapenem or meropenem). On discharge, fluoroquinolone or higher-generation cephalosporin with metronidazole, or amoxicillin-clavulanate are preferred oral (or parenteral) regimens. Most trials reported high antibiotic response rates, ranging from 88 to 100%. The duration of treatment for both intravenous and oral antibiotics was 7–10 days [12, 13].

There is no single approach to antibiotic therapy for uncomplicated acute appendicitis, and ongoing research and clinical trials continue to refine and validate effective regimens. Balancing the antibiotic spectrum, minimizing hospital stays, and tailoring treatment to individual patient needs remain key objectives in optimizing care for this condition.

2.2 Acute distended appendicitis (Mucocele of appendix)

Radiological imaging in patients with uncomplicated acute appendicitis may reveal a grossly distended appendix, filled with fluid, often due to obstruction or inflammation. The gross distention can be due to intraluminal accumulation of mucus. The management strategy involves a combination of antibiotic therapy and surgical intervention. Surgery is often necessary due to the high risk of progression to more severe complications such as perforation or abscess formation.

The gross distention in appendix can also arise from various other conditions, including retention cyst, mucosal hyperplasia, cystadenoma, and cystadenocarcinoma. Histopathological examination of the appendix, after surgical removal, may sometimes reveal low-grade mucinous neoplasm. Hence, one must be very cautious with these findings. The threshold for appendectomy should be very low to ensure that potential malignancies are not missed [14, 15].

The approach to surgery for appendiceal mucocele is guided by several key principles, which include resecting the appendix, performing a wide resection of the mesoappendix, and removing all associated lymph nodes to ensure complete clearance. The collected mucus should be analyzed cytologically to assess for malignant cells or other abnormalities. The base of the appendix should be carefully inspected to ensure no residual disease is left behind. More extensive surgical procedure such as right hemicolectomy or ileocecectomy is warranted to achieve complete tumor removal and prevent recurrence in positive margin at the base or positive peri appendiceal lymph nodes [16].

Complications like pseudomyxoma peritonei (PMP) can arise from the intraperitoneal rupture of an appendiceal mucinous neoplasm. To mitigate the risk of PMP, the surgery should be performed very cautiously to avoid perforation and spillage during removal [17].

In cases where the diagnosis is uncertain, maintaining a low threshold for surgical intervention is advisable.

2.3 Appendicolith

Approximately 25% of patients with appendicitis present with an appendicolith, a calcified deposit within the appendix (**Figures 1** and **2**). The presence of an appendicolith significantly influences the clinical course and management of appendicitis. Patients with imaging findings of appendicolith are at increased risk of complications, such as perforation and abscess formation. Additionally, patients with appendicolith experience higher failure rates with conservative treatment and have a greater likelihood of recurrence compared to those without appendicolith.

The CODA trial, which included patients with appendicoliths, provided insights into the clinical outcomes of appendicitis with appendicolith. In this study, 29% of patients in the antibiotics group required an appendectomy within 90 days, of which 41% had an appendicolith. The trial also highlighted that complications were predominantly associated with patients who had appendicoliths. These patients exhibited a higher risk of serious adverse events compared to those without appendicoliths [5].

In contrast, the APPAC trial, which excluded appendicoliths, reported less than 2% appendicular perforation among those who underwent appendectomy. On the other hand, the CODA trial, which included appendicoliths, found a significantly higher rate of appendiceal perforations at 16%, among which, 13% among those

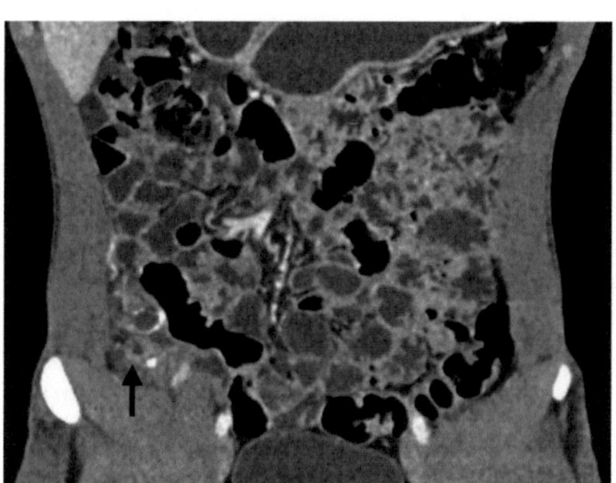

Figure 1.
CECT abdomen showing inflamed appendix with wall edema (arrow).

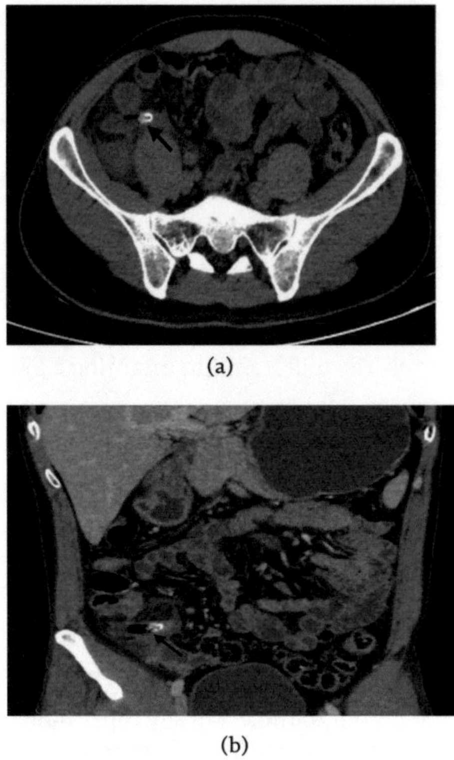

Figure 2.
Axial (a) and coronal (b) section CECT abdomen showing appendicolith (arrow) at base of perforated appendix with peri-appendiceal collection with air foci.

without an appendicolith. These findings underscore the impact of appendicoliths on appendiceal complications and management outcomes [3, 5].

Further investigation by Justin et al. investigated the feasibility of nonoperative management in children with acute appendicitis with an appendicolith identified on preoperative imaging. The failure rate of nonoperative management was 60% among the 14 children that were recruited, leading to the cessation of the study due to safety concerns [18].

Libin Huang et al. conducted a meta-analysis in children with uncomplicated appendicitis and compared antibiotic therapy with appendectomy. The analysis revealed a significantly increased risk for initial treatment failure and recurrent appendicitis in patients with appendicoliths, with a risk ratio of 10.43. In contrast, patients without appendicoliths had a lower risk of complications, with a risk ratio of 7.87 in the subgroup analysis [19].

The presence of appendicolith presents a major challenge in the management of acute appendicitis. An unacceptable high failure rate is seen among acute appendicitis patients with an appendicolith on nonoperative management, making early appendectomy the preferred approach to minimize complications and improve patient outcomes.

2.4 Recurrent appendicitis

Patients who initially receive nonoperative treatment for appendicitis may later present with recurrent episodes. It is essential to conduct a thorough evaluation of any

Uncomplicated appendicitis		
Types	**Preferred approach**	**Alternative option**
Acute catarrhal appendicitis	Antibiotic therapy	Operative intervention if conservative treatment fails
Acute distended appendicitis	Low threshold for surgery in view of risk of malignancy	Initial antibiotics followed by interval appendectomy
Appendicolith	Appendectomy, to prevent recurrence and other complications	Initial conservative management followed by interval appendectomy
Recurrent appendicitis	Operative treatment	Initial conservative if less severe or subacute infection, followed by interval appendectomy

Table 1.
Summary of treatment approach for uncomplicated appendicitis.

patient experiencing recurrent appendicitis to identify possible underlying issues, like missed appendicoliths or malignancy. Detailed assessment is crucial to uncover any predisposing factors or underlying conditions that could contribute to recurrence.

The debate between continuing nonoperative management and opting for appendectomy in cases of recurrent but uncomplicated appendicitis remains significant. According to the NOTA trial, among 159 patients who were managed nonoperatively with antibiotics, 11.9% were operated within 7 days, and the recurrence rates were noted to be 12.6% at 1 year and 13.8% at 2 years [20]. Similarly, the CODA trial revealed that among patients treated with antibiotics, 11% underwent appendectomy within 48 hours, 20% by 30 days, and 29% by 90 days [5]. The APPAC trial demonstrated that the incidence of appendectomy in the antibiotics group was 27% at 1 year, and 39% at 5 years [3]. These findings highlight the significant risk of recurrence following nonoperative management, particularly in patients with risk factors for appendicitis relapse. Therefore, patients with recurrent appendicitis, particularly those with underlying risk factors, should be considered for appendectomy to prevent further episodes and potential complications.

In some cases, patients with recurrent appendicitis may initially be managed with antibiotic therapy, particularly if the presentation is less severe and no evidence of complicated appendicitis is present. However, given the substantial risk of recurrence and the potential for increased complications, appendectomy remains a recommended option to ensure long-term resolution of appendicitis [21]. Treatment of various types of uncomplicated appendicitis is summarized in **Table 1**.

3. Complicated appendicitis

Complicated appendicitis includes a range of severe appendiceal conditions, including gangrene, perforation, peri appendiceal abscess and phlegmon formation. These complications require a meticulous treatment approach that integrates prompt diagnosis, effective antibiotic therapy, and often, surgical intervention. These patients are acutely ill, and initial resuscitation and antibiotics play a critical role in treatment.

The definite management strategy for complicated appendicitis depends on the hemodynamic stability of patient and the nature of perforation, whether it is contained or free. The presence of an abscess or phlegmon, as indicated by imaging studies, also plays a significant role in guiding treatment decisions.

In general, if the patient is hemodynamically unstable, immediate surgical intervention is indicated. In such cases, urgent appendectomy is necessary to address the source of infection and prevent further deterioration. If patients are stable, initial management can begin with conservative measures. This includes the administration of intravenous antibiotics, fluid resuscitation, and bowel rest. Close monitoring is essential during the initial phase of treatment. The stabilization of patient and control of infection are the primary goals of this nonoperative management. If the patient's condition does not worsen, an interval appendectomy may be planned at a later stage [22, 23]. This approach allows time for inflammation to subside and the patient to recover from the acute phase. Improvement in symptoms, such as a reduction in fever, tenderness, and leukocytosis, generally allows for a gradual advancement of diet, typically within 3–5 days. Once stabilized and clinical parameters normalize, patients are discharged. Follow-up visits are scheduled for 6–8 weeks post-discharge to monitor recovery and plan for interval appendectomy. If a patient shows signs of treatment failure, such as bowel obstruction, sepsis or pain, fever, or leukocytosis, prompt surgical intervention is warranted. Delayed surgical intervention can be beneficial, as it is associated with a reduced need for extensive appendectomy resections, reduced operative duration, and a tendency toward reduced mortality rates.

The choice of antibiotics for complicated appendicitis is continuously evolving and varies according to hemodynamic condition and severity of infection. Empiric antibiotic therapy should address a wide range of pathogens, including gram-negative rods and anaerobic bacteria. Recent guidelines recommend broad-spectrum regimens, such as piperacillin-tazobactam or carbapenems, to effectively target the diverse bacterial flora associated with complicated appendicitis [24].

3.1 Perforated or gangrenous appendicitis

In unstable patients with free perforation or gangrenous appendicitis, generalized peritonitis is usually present. Immediate surgical intervention is crucial in such cases. The initial step involves resuscitation with intravenous fluids to address dehydration and stabilize hemodynamically, along with prompt administration of broad-spectrum antibiotics. An immediate appendectomy is required, along with thorough drainage and irrigation of peritoneal cavity to manage the infection and prevent further complications.

The choice between open or laparoscopic approach depends on surgeon's expertize, the patient's condition, and available resources. If open approach is chosen, the procedure may be done through local site incisions (as explained later) or a midline laparotomy, depending upon the degree of peritoneal contamination and patient's systemic status. This should be followed by an antibiotic course of 5–7 days based on culture reports and the patient's response [25].

Current guidelines suggest that surgery for perforated appendicitis should be performed as early as possible, preferentially within 8 hours of diagnosis, to mitigate the risk of severe complications and improve patient outcomes. However, recent studies suggest that in clinically stable patients with symptoms localized to the right iliac fossa, initial nonoperative management with close monitoring can be a safe option. These patients may undergo interval appendectomy 4–6 weeks later, once the local inflammatory process has resolved. The timing of surgery in such cases is ultimately at the discretion of the treating surgeon, as no study with strong recommendations are available to provide specific guidelines [26].

Postoperatively, intravenous antibiotic therapy is continued. Patient should be monitored for signs of wound infection or intra-abdominal abscess formation. Ensuring adequate pain control, early mobilization, and nutritional support are also crucial aspects of postoperative care.

3.2 Appendicular abscess

The management of appendiceal abscess can be approached either operatively or conservatively. Immediate appendectomy may be technically demanding due to extensive inflammation, potentially leading to extensive resections. Therefore, conservative management initially followed by interval appendectomy is often considered the gold standard.

The initial assessment of the abscess should determine whether it is amenable to percutaneous drainage. Treatment strategy for abscesses more than 3 cm should involve a combination of systemic antibiotic therapy and image-guided percutaneous drainage initially. The procedure can be performed under ultrasound or CT guidance or therapeutic aspiration may suffice. An appropriate course of intravenous antibiotics is administered. If percutaneous drainage is not feasible and conservative treatment fails, the patient will need to undergo an appendectomy during the same hospital admission [27].

Evidence indicates that managing appendicular abscesses through percutaneous drainage generally yields more favorable outcomes and has a shorter hospital stay and reduced complication rates. This approach allows inflammation to diminish prior to appendectomy, potentially reducing the need for more extensive bowel resections such as ileocecectomy. A meta-analysis by Similis et al., which included 17 randomized and non-randomized studies, demonstrated that immediate appendectomy is associated with significantly higher rates of complications including intestinal obstruction, deep abdominal or pelvic abscesses, and wound infections [28]. These results were corroborated by the meta-analysis by Vaos et al. and by other studies [29–31]. However, there are few studies showing contradictory results. In a retrospective study conducted by Young et al., early appendectomy proved to be more effective than initial nonoperative management for appendicular abscesses. Out of 95 patients, 60 had an early appendectomy, while 35 initially received nonoperative management. Among those who failed nonoperative management, 25.7% required open surgery, with most needing bowel resection. The study concluded that early appendectomy was associated with a significantly lower rate of extensive bowel resection (3.3% compared to 17.1%, $P = 0.048$) compared to patients who were managed conservatively initially [32].

Sadozai L et al. analyzed several factors predicting the response to conservative management like the trend of CRP and the white blood cells, presence of multiple abscesses or stercolith. The study concluded that patients with multiple abscesses should not be treated with antibiotics alone [33].

The necessity for appendectomy following successful initial conservative management remains a topic of debate. Given the potential for underlying conditions such as cancer or recurrent disease, the decision to proceed with appendectomy should be carefully considered. For patients who are not scheduled for an appendectomy, it is crucial to conduct thorough screening to rule out other serious conditions. This involves a colonoscopy or CT scan of the abdomen to detect any possible underlying pathology such as malignancy or other gastrointestinal disorders. Additionally, patients should be under careful surveillance to monitor for any signs of disease recurrence or progression [12].

3.3 Phlegmon

The ideal treatment protocol for complicated appendicitis with phlegmon is a subject of ongoing discussion. Traditionally, immediate appendectomy in phlegmon is often associated with higher morbidity and complications and may not be feasible due to extensive inflammation. If the patient responds well to initial antibiotic therapy and is hemodynamically stable, conservative management with oral or intravenous antibiotics for 7–10 days is recommended, followed by a planned interval appendectomy later. This approach allows local inflammation to decrease and performing appendectomy at a lower risk. According to a 2010 meta-analysis of 17 non-randomized trials, initial nonoperative management results in fewer complications, comparable period of hospitalization, and duration of antibiotics in perforated appendix with abscess or phlegmon [28].

For patients presenting with hemodynamic instability or those who do not improve with antibiotics, surgery is necessary. Due to dense adhesions, appendectomy can be challenging, often requiring ileocecal resection and leading to higher morbidity. Under these circumstances, extensive dissection may cause injury of adjacent structures, resulting in complications like postoperative abscess or enterocutaneous fistulas, which might require further surgery such as ileocolectomy or cecectomy [34].

Laparoscopic surgery, in experienced hands, is safe and feasible and has shown to be associated with fewer hospital admissions and additional intervention than conservative management. If laparoscopic expertize is available, it can also be considered a first-line management for both phlegmon and appendicular abscesses. Nonoperative management remains a rational initial line treatment approach for appendicitis presenting with phlegmon.

Recurrence rates after non-surgical management for appendiceal abscesses range from 12 to 24%. Routine interval appendectomy after nonoperative management is not recommended for young adults and children due to its cost-effectiveness and limited benefit. It should be reserved for those with recurring symptoms [35]. For patients over 40, who have a higher risk of appendiceal neoplasms, both colonoscopy and contrast-enhanced CT scans are advised for thorough evaluation [36]. The treatment approaches for complicated appendicitis are summarized in **Table 2**.

Complicated appendicitis		
Types	**Preferred approach**	**Alternative option**
Perforated/ gangrenous appendicitis	Early operative intervention.	In stable patients, trial of initial conservative management followed by interval appendectomy.
Appendicular abscess	Image guided percutaneous drainage of abscess ± interval appendectomy.	Surgical drainage with appendectomy (if abscess not drainable or failed conservative therapy).
Phlegmon	Initial antibiotic therapy, followed by planned interval appendectomy later.	Operative intervention if hemodynamically unstable, or failed initial conservative approach.

Table 2.
Treatment approach for complicated appendicitis.

4. Appendicitis in special population

4.1 Pregnancy

Acute appendicitis is the most common non-obstetric, surgical emergency during pregnancy, and can occur in any trimester. Early diagnosis and intervention are essential to avoid potential life-threatening complications for both mother and fetus. Non-surgical management with antibiotics alone is associated with poorer outcomes during pregnancy, making appendectomy the preferred treatment option [37].

Appendectomy can be done by laparoscopic or open approach. According to the Society of American Gastrointestinal and Endoscopic Surgeons (SAGES), laparoscopic appendectomy is considered safe throughout all trimesters and is standard of care [38]. The choice between laparoscopic and open surgery depends on factors such as the patient's clinical status, gestational age, and size of gravid uterus. The laparoscopic approach is generally preferred as it facilitates the identification of variable localization of the appendix and allows to evaluate the whole abdomen for other ongoing pathological process. However, some studies suggest that laparoscopic surgery may have a higher risk of fetal loss. Modifications for laparoscopic appendectomy during pregnancy include positioning the patient slightly left-lateral after 20 weeks of gestation to reduce venacaval compression, using an open-access technique for first trocar, limiting intraabdominal pressure to 12 mm Hg, and adjusting port sites according to the size of the uterus [39, 40].

For open appendectomy, a transverse incision is made at the point of maximum tenderness, not necessarily at McBurney's point. If the diagnosis is uncertain, a lower midline incision can be used to expose the abdomen and access other surgical conditions that may mimic appendicitis. In cases of appendiceal perforation, if it is not contained, an urgent laparotomy for appendectomy with irrigation and drainage of the peritoneal cavity is necessary [41]. For contained perforation presenting late, conservative management with antibiotics, intravenous fluids, and bowel rest may be appropriate. Immediate surgery in these patients is associated with increased morbidity due to adhesions and inflammation and unavoidable injury to adjacent structures [37]. Careful monitoring in the hospital is essential to prevent complications such as sepsis, preterm labor, or fetal loss.

There is limited evidence on the interventional drainage of appendiceal abscesses in pregnant patients. A study by Matthew et al., which analyzed 8087 pregnant women with complicated appendicitis, found that only 11% could be successfully managed conservatively. The study also indicated that immediate appendectomy was linked to fewer maternal infectious complications and no increased risk of preterm delivery, preterm labor, abortion, or antepartum hemorrhage [42].

4.2 Older patients

Due to diminished inflammatory response in older adults, these patients present with less pronounced symptoms and findings on history and examination. Consequently, these patients are more likely to present late with complicated appendicitis. Additionally, the presence of multiple comorbid conditions in this age group can increase both perioperative morbidity and mortality [43, 44].

Older adults are also at a higher risk of having occult appendiceal malignancies. According to the "Surveillance, Epidemiology, and End Results (SEER)" review database from 2000 to 2014, 28.6% of appendiceal cancers in individuals over 65 years were initially misdiagnosed as acute appendicitis [45]. To enhance diagnostic accuracy in this population, CT scans are useful. Additionally, patients aged more than 40 years who receive conservative treatment should undergo a colonoscopy and should be evaluated for an interval appendectomy [36]. If these patients are planned for conservative management, it should be approached with caution, incorporating radiological imaging in follow-up and interval appendectomy as a part of the treatment strategy.

4.3 Immunocompromised

Due to the blunted immune response, these patients are at higher risk of infection including opportunistic or viral infection and fungal infections and may not present with the typical signs and symptoms. The diagnosis becomes difficult as they might not show the expected level of inflammatory changes in laboratory and radiological tests. The differential diagnosis can include a range of conditions such as opportunistic infections (e.g., mycobacterial), viral (e.g., cytomegalovirus), and fungal infections or secondary malignancies (e.g., lymphoma, Kaposi's sarcoma). This wide array of possible diseases delays accurate diagnosis and therefore delaying surgical evaluation, which raises the risk of perforation [46]. If there is a strong suspicion of appendicitis, the threshold for surgical intervention should be less, as there are no specific contraindications to surgery for immunocompromised patients and nonoperative management has not been well researched in this group.

5. Surgical aspects

Appendectomy remains one of the most commonly performed surgeries around the world. It is a relatively safe procedure, with overall mortality of 0.09–0.24% [47]. Open and laparoscopic are the two most commonly used approaches to perform appendectomy, with other few novel minimally invasive approaches. In recent years, laparoscopic surgery has surpassed the frequency of open appendectomy in both complicated and uncomplicated appendicitis. Laparoscopic surgery is associated with decreased wound infection rates, shorter hospital stay, lesser postoperative pain, decreased postoperative wound infections, and earlier postoperative recovery. Patients with diffuse peritonitis may require a lower midline laparotomy incision to allow thorough peritoneal irrigation. In this section, various surgical aspects of these different approaches will be discussed.

5.1 Preoperative preparations

The patient should be adequately hydrated and resuscitated before taking up for surgery. Like any other abdominal surgery, antibiotic prophylaxis should be given prior to surgery, preferably within 30–60 minutes of incision. Generally, antibiotics with broad coverage are indicated to reduce the chances of intra-abdominal abscesses or SSI in the postoperative period. A nasogastric tube and Foley catheterization may be required in cases with generalized peritonitis and unstable clinical conditions.

5.2 Open appendectomy

Open appendectomy is generally performed via the local site incisions. Access to the appendix can be achieved via the oblique incision (McBurney's incision) at

McBurney's point or transverse incision (Rockey-Davis incision). The McBurney's incision is made perpendicular to the spino-umbilical line at 1/3rd distance from the right anterior superior iliac spine. Lanz incision is a modification of McBurney's incision and is more cosmetic and made along the Langer's line. Rockey-Davis incision is a horizontal incision and can be extended medially (Fowler Weir extension) or laterally (Rutherford Morrison extension) for better exposure (**Figure 3**).

The abdominal wall muscles (external oblique, internal oblique, and transversus abdominis) are separated along its fibers using blunt dissection to reach the peritoneum. The peritoneum is lifted between two artery forceps and sharply cut to enter the abdomen. The first step is to locate the appendix. We attempt to visualize the cecum first and follow the taenia till the confluence to reach the appendiceal base. Appendix is freed from surrounding adhesions by blunt dissection and is delivered outside through the incision grasping with Babcock forceps. Window is created between the mesoappendix and the base of the appendix using a right-angle forceps. The base is then crushed using medium artery forceps and ligated distally with an absorbable suture (**Figure 4**). Appendix is then divided proximal to the artery forceps, and the stump mucosa is burnt using electrocautery. The mesoappendix is dissected, and the appendicular artery is clamped between two hemostats, divided, and suture ligated (**Figure 5**). Peritoneum and fascial layers are closed. Skin is approximated using sutures or staplers [48].

Leaving the skin open in heavily contaminated cases like perforated or gangrenous appendicitis has been practiced at some centers. However, recent studies recommend primary wound closure with antibiotic coverage even in class III or IV surgery [49]. The open approach of appendectomy is preferred in the absence of well-trained assistants or unavailability of the laparoscopic facility. The laparoscopic approach has surpassed the open approach in all aspects and has added benefits over the open technique as discussed in the next section.

5.3 Laparoscopic appendectomy

Laparoscopic approach is both safe and effective for uncomplicated appendicitis, even in complicated appendicitis based on the surgeon's experience. Another advantage of laparoscopic surgery is its ability to correctly confirm other diagnoses which may mimic appendicitis and proceed with laparoscopic management for the same.

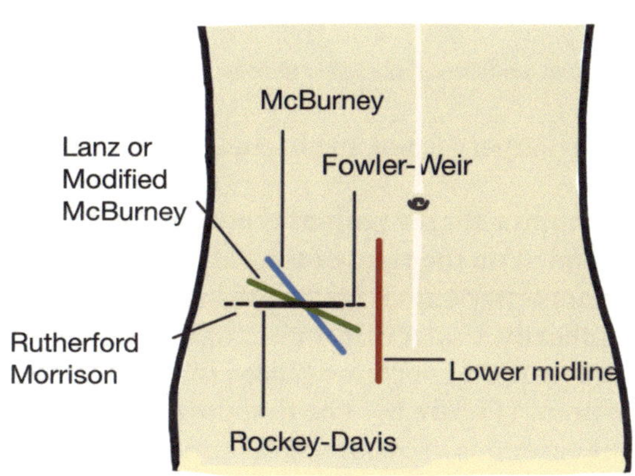

Figure 3.
Various incisions used for open appendectomy.

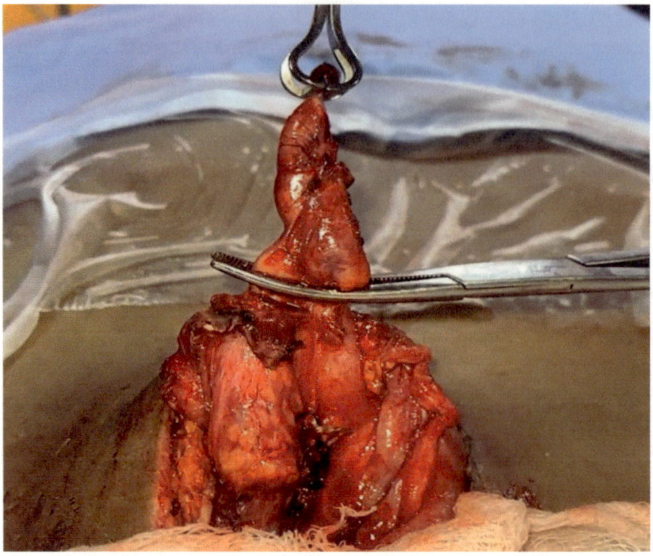

Figure 4.
Base of the appendix was crushed using a hemostat forceps.

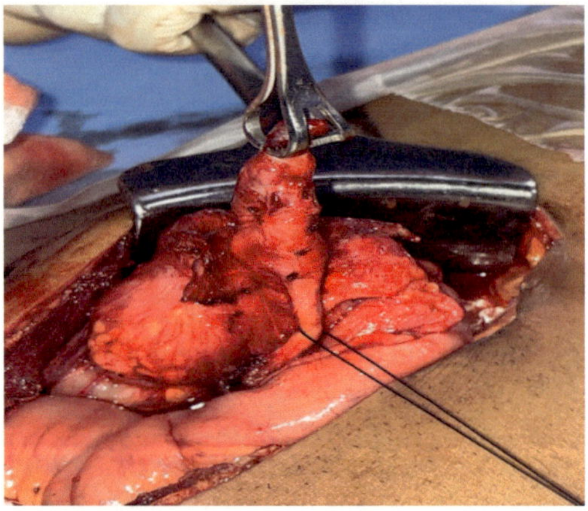

Figure 5.
Appendicular artery looped around a silk thread through a window in the mesoappendix.

Previous open abdominal surgery is not an absolute contraindication for laparoscopic appendectomy.

For the laparoscopic approach, the patient is positioned supine with arms tucked in. The monitor is positioned on the right of the patient, and the surgeon stands on the left. Initially, pneumoperitoneum is created using open Hassen's technique or Veress needle peri-umbilically. Under direct visualization using a laparoscope (5 or 10 mm), two other 5 mm working ports are placed in the midline in suprapubic position and left lower quadrant (**Figure 6**). The first port is used to grasp and manipulate the appendix, while the second is used for the operating instruments. A third trocar may be required based on intraoperative findings, like in cases of densely adherent appendix or a long subhepatic appendix. After ports are placed, Trendelenburg position with right side tilted up provides better visibility of appendix [50, 51].

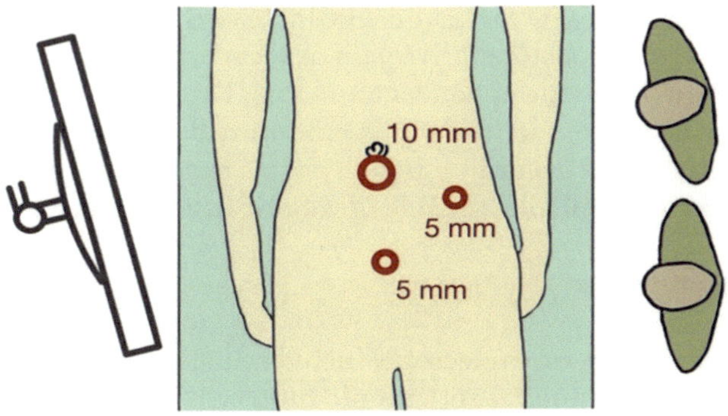

Figure 6.
Operating room setup for laparoscopic appendectomy with the surgeon standing on the left of the patient and monitor on the right. Traditional three-port sites for laparoscopic appendectomy are also shown.

After positioning and diagnostic laparoscopy, the overlying omentum and small bowel are swiped away cranially. The terminal ileum and ileocecal junction are identified, and cecum is traced. In normal anatomy, the appendicular base is visualized at the confluence of three taenia. Rarely, mobilization of caecum and ascending colon may be required for visualization of the appendicular base. Once visualized, the appendix is grasped from its tip or body and held taut to visualize the mesoappendix. The mesoappendix is divided using bipolar cautery till its base and artery is ligated using a vascular stapler or clip. It is advised to avoid monopolar cautery due to the chances of injury to bowel or adjacent structures. In cases of perforated appendicitis, extra caution is exercised when handling tissues. Any adhesions due to inflammation can be separated by blunt and sharp dissection, if necessary, and the use of monopolar cautery is discouraged [51]. A window is created between the mesoappendix and the base of appendix using Maryland dissector. Linear stapling devices or suture snares are used to divide the appendix at its base. If the base is inflamed or perforated, a cuff of cecum may have to be removed by placing the stapler slightly higher. Resected appendix is retrieved in endoscopic bag through the 10 mm umbilical port. Fascial closure is done for 10 mm port to prevent the port site hernia [48].

If dense adhesions or technical difficulties prevent safe removal of the appendix through a laparoscopic approach, a decision to switch to open should be made. The conversion rate varies widely, from 0 to 27%, largely depending on the surgeon's exposure to the procedure [52].

5.4 Robotic appendectomy

Robotic appendectomy, despite being a safe and having equal efficacy comparable to the laparoscopic approach, has not yet achieved widespread adoption in clinical practice. The robotic approach improves the precision of surgery, visualization, and dexterity and reduces tremors. It also makes remote surgery possible. These benefits have led to the adoption of robotic systems in complex abdominal procedures [53].

For appendectomy, studies comparing laparoscopic and robotic approach have indicated that the operative time, length of hospital stay, and complication rates are comparable and fall within acceptable clinical parameters [53, 54]. The surgical principles and operative steps remain the same with conventional approaches, after initial docking of the robotic system.

Despite the advantages, several factors like increased cost, limited ability, and lack of clear superiority in postoperative pain or recovery duration have limited the widespread adoption of robotic appendectomy [55]. Laparoscopic appendectomy remains the gold standard modality for this procedure due to the absence of definitive advantages. As refinements occur in robotic systems to address current limitations, and more data becomes available, the role of robotic in appendectomy may evolve.

5.5 Other novel techniques

Advanced techniques in appendectomy include single port laparoscopic appendectomy, natural orifice transluminal endoscopic surgery (NOTES)-appendectomy with its different variations.

Single-port laparoscopic appendectomy has emerged as a viable approach and has nearly comparable patient satisfaction and safety as compared to conventional three-port laparoscopic surgery. This technique has not gained widespread, most likely due to the requirement for specialized training and equipment. Studies have failed to establish the superiority of single-port approach over the laparoscopic approach [56, 57].

NOTES-appendectomy represents the cutting edge of minimally invasive surgical techniques for appendectomy. Transgastric and transvaginal approaches for intraperitoneal access have been explored for appendectomy so far. The approach is still experimental, and more prospective randomized trials are required to standardize this technique. NOTES aims to further reduce surgical trauma and improve cosmetic outcomes compared to traditional laparoscopic approaches [56].

5.6 Postoperative complications

Over the past decades, surgical techniques have evolved from open appendectomy to laparoscopic appendectomy and more recently to robotic-assisted appendectomy. Multiple studies and meta-analyses have consistently shown lower overall complication rates for laparoscopic appendectomy compared to open approach, particularly for wound infections. Robotic appendectomy appears to have comparable or slightly lower complication rates than laparoscopic appendectomy [58, 59].

5.6.1 Wound infection

Superficial or deep SSI may occur within 30 days of appendectomy and present with incisional pain, wound discharge or fever. There may be associated wound dehiscence or positive wound culture [60]. Compared to laparoscopic appendectomy, open appendectomy is prone to higher risk of incision site infection, (4.6 vs. 11% per 100 appendectomies) [61].

The SSI rates can be reduced by meticulous skin preparation before surgery, antibiotic prophylaxis within 60 minutes of incision, sterile technique, and appropriate antibiotic coverage postoperatively. Early recognition of signs and symptoms can prevent the spread to deeper tissue and reduce wound morbidity. Treatment involves wound care, antimicrobial therapy based on culture results and debridement as and when required.

5.6.2 Intra-abdominal abscess

Pelvic abscess may develop in up to 9.4% of post-appendectomy patients [62]. This complication can be prevented by thorough peritoneal irrigation adequate drainage and culture-guided antibiotic therapy postoperatively. Laparoscopic appendectomy showed a higher frequency of this complication (6.4%) compared to open approach (3%) [63]. However, recent studies suggest that the technique of appendectomy does not affect the incidence of postoperative intra-abdominal abscess [64].

Intra-abdominal abscess is initially managed with image-guided drainage or aspiration along with broad-spectrum antibiotics. However, surgical intervention may be necessary for patients having persistent fever and pain unresponsive to conservative treatment, or those with multiple abscess pockets.

5.6.3 Stump appendicitis

Stump appendicitis is a rare form of recurrent appendicitis in the long remnant stump and can happen after open or laparoscopic appendectomy, with incidence of 1 in 50,000 cases [65]. This occurs most commonly in cases of perforated appendicitis [66]. It may present with classical symptoms of acute appendicitis or with non-specific chronic abdominal pain. Diagnosis can be confirmed by USG or CT scan showing tubular remnant arising from the base of cecum with inflammatory changes and surrounding collection.

Surgical removal of remnant stump remains the standard treatment for stump appendicitis, either via open or laparoscopic approach. A perforated appendiceal stump or involvement of cecum, or suspicion of malignancy, may require a more extensive bowel resection. To reduce this risk, resection of sufficient appendiceal tissue with less than 5 mm of stump preservation is advised [67].

5.6.4 Fecal fistula

Fecal fistula is a rare occurrence and presents with distressing symptoms. It typically originates from appendiceal stump. This may occur in cases with severe peri-appendiceal inflammation, technical errors like injury to cecum during appendectomy or in patients with underlying malignancy, tuberculosis or Crohn's disease.

Treatment may be conservative or surgical. Most of these fecal fistulae respond well to conservative treatment including drainage of any collection and antibiotic therapy, in the absence of underlying disease. If conservative treatment fails or suspicion of underlying condition is there, fistula excision with segmental bowel resection is recommended [68].

5.6.5 Ventral hernia

Incisional hernia, though infrequent (0.4–0.9%), is a potential complication following open appendectomy. It typically develops at the site of the McBurney incision, due to weakening of the abdominal wall attributed to ilio-inguinal or ilio-hypogastric nerves injury during the surgery. Other risk factors include obesity, wound infection, and poor wound healing [69].

Management options range from watchful waiting for asymptomatic cases to surgical repair, with techniques including primary closure, mesh reinforcement, or laparoscopic approaches [70]. The choice of intervention depends on hernia size, patient factors, and surgeon expertize. Preventive strategies include meticulous closure techniques, infection control, and optimizing patient-related risk factors preoperatively.

6. Conclusion

The management of appendicitis has evolved significantly, with treatment strategies now tailored to the specific presentation—uncomplicated or complicated. For uncomplicated cases, antibiotic therapy has emerged as a viable alternative to surgery in selected patients, though the risk of recurrence remains a concern. Complicated appendicitis, including perforated, gangrenous, or abscess-forming cases, often requires a combination of antibiotics and surgical intervention. The approach may be immediate surgery or initial conservative management followed by interval appendectomy, depending on the patient's condition and local expertize. Ongoing research continues to refine treatment protocols, aiming to optimize outcomes while minimizing unnecessary interventions.

Conflict of interest

Authors declare no conflict of interest.

Author details

Summi Karn, Navin Kumar*, Karamveer Singh and Somprakas Basu
All India Institute of Medical Sciences, Rishikesh, India

*Address all correspondence to: navin.surg@aiimsrishikesh.edu.in

IntechOpen

© 2024 The Author(s). Licensee IntechOpen. This chapter is distributed under the terms of the Creative Commons Attribution License (http://creativecommons.org/licenses/by/4.0), which permits unrestricted use, distribution, and reproduction in any medium, provided the original work is properly cited.

References

[1] Hamill JK, Hill AG. A history of the treatment of appendicitis in children: Lessons learned. ANZ Journal of Surgery. 2016;**86**(9):730-735. DOI: 10.1111/ans.13627

[2] Bom WJ, Scheijmans JCG, Salminen P, Boermeester MA. Diagnosis of uncomplicated and complicated appendicitis in adults. Scandinavian Journal of Surgery. 2021;**110**(2):170-179. DOI: 10.1177/14574969211008330

[3] Salminen P, Tuominen R, Paajanen H, et al. Five-year follow-up of antibiotic therapy for uncomplicated acute appendicitis in the APPAC randomized clinical trial. Journal of the American Medical Association. 2018;**320**(12):1259-1265. DOI: 10.1001/jama.2018.13201

[4] Rollins KE, Verinder J, Bedrebo D, et al. Antibiotics versus appendicectomy for the treatment of uncomplicated acute appendicitis: An updated meta-analysis of randomized controlled trials. World Journal of Surgery. 2016;**40**(10):2305-2318. DOI: 10.1007/s00268-016-3561-7

[5] The CODA Collaborative. A randomized trial comparing antibiotics with appendectomy for appendicitis. The New England Journal of Medicine. 2020;**383**(20):1907-1919. DOI: 10.1056/NEJMoa2014320

[6] Chen CY, Chen YC, Pu HN, et al. Bacteriology of acute appendicitis and its implication for the use of prophylactic antibiotics. Surgical Infections. 2012;**13**(6):383-390. DOI: 10.1089/sur.2016.261

[7] Mazuski JE, Solomkin JS, Bradley JS, et al. The surgical infection society revised guidelines on the management of intra-abdominal infection. Surgical Infections. 2017;**18**(1):1-76. DOI: 10.1089/sur.2016.261

[8] Solomkin JS, Mazuski JE, Bradley JS, et al. Diagnosis and management of complicated intra-abdominal infection in adults and children: Guidelines by the surgical infection society and the Infectious Diseases Society of America. Clinical Infectious Diseases. 2010;**50**(2):133-164. DOI: 10.1086/649554

[9] De Waele JJ, Tellado JM, Alder J, et al. Randomised clinical trial of moxifloxacin versus ertapenem in complicated intra-abdominal infections: Results of the PROMISE study. International Journal of Antimicrobial Agents. 2013;**41**(1):57-64. DOI: 10.1016/j.ijantimicag.2012.09.017

[10] Goldstein EJ, Solomkin JS, Citron DM, et al. Clinical efficacy and correlation of clinical outcomes with in vitro susceptibility for anaerobic bacteria in patients with complicated intra-abdominal infections treated with moxifloxacin. Clinical Infectious Diseases. 2011;**53**(11):1074-1080. DOI: 10.1093/cid/cir672

[11] Haijanen J, Salminen P, Grönroos JM, et al. Optimising the antibiotic treatment of uncomplicated acute appendicitis: A protocol for a multicentre randomised clinical trial (APPAC II trial). BMJ Open. 2017;**7**(8):117. DOI: 10.1136/bmjopen-2016-015348

[12] Di Saverio S, Birindelli A, Kelly MD, et al. WSES Jerusalem guidelines for diagnosis and treatment of acute appendicitis. World Journal of Emergency Surgery: WJES. 2016;**11**:34. DOI: 10.1186/s13017-016-0090-5

[13] Talan DA, Saltzman DJ, DeUgarte DA, Moran GJ. Methods of

conservative antibiotic treatment of acute uncomplicated appendicitis: A systematic review. Journal of Trauma and Acute Care Surgery. 2019;**86**(4):722-736. DOI: 10.1097/TA.0000000000002137

[14] Rabie ME, Fagihi A, Al Shammari M, et al. Mucus-containing cystic lesions "mucocele" of the appendix: The unresolved issues. International Journal of Surgical Oncology. 2015;**2015**:139461. DOI: 10.1155/2015/139461

[15] Saad EA, Elsamani EY, AbdElrahim WE, et al. Surgical treatment of mucocele of the appendix: a systematic review and case report. Journal of Surgical Case Reports. 2018;**2018**(6):rjy102. DOI: 10.1093/jscr/rjy102

[16] Dhage-Ivatury S, Sugarbaker PH. Update on the surgical approach to mucocele of the appendix. Journal of the American College of Surgeons. 2006;**202**(4):680-684. DOI: 10.1016/j.jamcollsurg.2005.12.003

[17] Misdraji J. Mucinous epithelial neoplasms of the appendix and pseudomyxoma peritonei. Modern Pathology. 2015;**28**(Suppl):1-79. DOI: 10.1038/modpathol.2014.129

[18] Mahida JB, Lodwick DL, Nacion KM, et al. High failure rate of nonoperative management of acute appendicitis with an appendicolith in children. Journal of Pediatric Surgery. 2016;**51**(6):908-911. DOI: 10.1016/j.jpedsurg.2016.02.056

[19] Huang L, Yin Y, Yang L, et al. Comparison of antibiotic therapy and appendectomy for acute uncomplicated appendicitis in children: A meta-analysis. JAMA Pediatrics. 2017;**171**(5):426-434. DOI: 10.1001/jamapediatrics.2017.0057

[20] Di Saverio S, Podda M, De Simone B, et al. The NOTA study (non operative treatment for acute appendicitis): Prospective study on the efficacy and safety of antibiotics for treating patients with right lower quadrant abdominal pain and long-term follow-up of conservatively treated suspected appendicitis. Annals of Surgery. 2014;**260**(1):109-117. DOI: 10.1097/SLA.0000000000000560

[21] Flum DR, Collaborative CODA. Factors associated with recurrent appendicitis after successful treatment with antibiotics. The British Journal of Surgery. 2023;**110**(11):1482-1489. DOI: 10.1093/bjs/znad218

[22] Zhou S, Cheng Y, Cheng N, et al. Early versus delayed appendicectomy for appendiceal phlegmon or abscess. Cochrane Database of Systematic Reviews. 2024;**5**(5):CD011670. DOI: 10.1002/14651858.CD011670.pub3

[23] Oliak D, Yamini D, Udani VM, et al. Initial nonoperative management for periappendiceal abscess. Diseases of the Colon and Rectum. 2001;**44**(7):936-941. DOI: 10.1007/BF02235479

[24] Smith J, Brown A. Empirical antibiotic therapy for complicated appendicitis: A review of current practices. World Journal of Surgical Infection. 2021;**15**(3):245-258. DOI: 10.1016/j.surg.2021.01.005

[25] Balogun OS, Osinowo A, Afolayan M, et al. Acute perforated appendicitis in adults: Management and complications in Lagos, Nigeria. Annals of African Medicine. 2019;**18**(1):36-41. DOI: 10.4103/aam.aam_11_18

[26] Calpin GG, Hembrecht S, Giblin K, et al. The impact of timing on outcomes in appendicectomy: A systematic review and network meta-analysis. World Journal of Emergency Surgery: WJES. 2024;**19**(1):24. DOI: 10.1186/s13017-024-00549-4

[27] Rosenblum D. Management of acute appendicitis in adults. In: UpToDate [Internet]. Waltham (MA): UpToDate; 2024. Available from: https://www.uptodate.com/contents/management-of-acute-appendicitis-in-adults

[28] Simillis C, Symeonides P, Shorthouse AJ, Tekkis PP. A meta-analysis comparing conservative treatment versus acute appendectomy for complicated appendicitis (abscess or phlegmon). Surgery. 2010;**147**(6):818-829. DOI: 10.1016/j.surg.2009.11.013

[29] Demetrashvili Z, Kenchadze G, Pipia I, et al. Comparison of treatment methods of appendiceal mass and abscess: A prospective cohort study. Annals of Medicine and Surgery. 2019;**48**:48-52. DOI: 10.1016/j.amsu.2019.10.002

[30] Erdoğan D, Karaman I, Narci A, et al. Comparison of two methods for the management of appendicular mass in children. Pediatric Surgery International. 2005;**21**(2):81-83. DOI: 10.1007/s00383-004-1334-0

[31] Perez KS, Allen SR. Complicated appendicitis and considerations for interval appendectomy. JAAPA. 2018;**31**(9):35-41. DOI: 10.1097/01.JAA.0000544295.37330.50

[32] Young KA, Neuhaus NM, Fluck M, et al. Outcomes of complicated appendicitis: Is conservative management as smooth as it seems? American Journal of Surgery. 2018;**215**(4):586-592. DOI: 10.1016/j.amjsurg.2017.10.032

[33] Sadozai L, Chouikh T, Kotobi H, et al. Optimization of the medical management of appendicular abscess and plastron in children: A 2009 to 2019 cohort study. Clinical Research. 2023;**8**:3642. DOI: 10.21203/rs.3.rs-1975554/v1

[34] De Almeida Leite RM, Lopes LR, Kallas DM, et al. Delayed operative management in complicated acute appendicitis—Is avoiding extended resection worth the wait? Results from a global cohort study. Journal of Gastrointestinal Surgery. 2022;**26**(7):1482-1489. DOI: 10.1007/s11605-022-05311-2

[35] Bendib H. Is non-operative treatment of acute appendicitis possible: A narrative review. African Journal of Emergency Medicine. 2024;**14**(2):84-90. DOI: 10.1016/j.afjem.2024.03.006

[36] Carpenter SG, Ng Y, Heil EL, et al. Increased risk of neoplasm in appendicitis treated with interval appendectomy: Single-institution experience and literature review. The American Surgeon. 2012;**78**(3):339-343. DOI: 10.1177/000313481207800312

[37] Aptilon Duque G, Oladipo AF, Lotfollahzadeh S. Appendicitis in pregnancy. In: StatPearls [Internet]. Treasure Island (FL): StatPearls Publishing; 2024. Available from: https://www.ncbi.nlm.nih.gov/books/NBK551642/

[38] Pearl JP, Price RR, Tonkin AE, Richardson WS, Stefanidis D. SAGES guidelines for the use of laparoscopy during pregnancy. Surgical Endoscopy. 2017;**31**(10):3767-3782. DOI: 10.1007/s00464-017-5637-3

[39] Korndorffer JR, Fellinger E, Reed W. SAGES guideline for laparoscopic appendectomy. Surgical Endoscopy. 2010;**24**(4):757-761. DOI: 10.1007/s00464-009-0651-2

[40] Walker HG, Al Samaraee A, Mills SJ, Kalbassi MR. Laparoscopic appendicectomy in pregnancy: A systematic review of the published evidence. International Journal of

Surgery. 2014;**12**(11):1235-1241. DOI: 10.1016/j.ijsu.2014.08.354

[41] Hodjati H, Kazerooni T. Location of the appendix in the gravid patient: A re-evaluation of the established concept. International Journal of Gynaecology and Obstetrics. 2003;**81**(3):245-247. DOI: 10.1016/S0020-7292(03)00077-2

[42] Ashbrook M, Cheng V, Sandhu K, et al. Management of complicated appendicitis during pregnancy in the US. JAMA Netw Open. 2022;**5**(4):e227555. DOI:10.1001/jamanetworkopen.2022.7555

[43] Watters JM, Blakslee JM, March RJ, Redmond ML. The influence of age on the severity of peritonitis. Canadian Journal of Surgery. 1996;**39**(2):142-146. DOI: 10.1503/cjs.0392142

[44] Fan SM, Grigorian A, Smith BR, et al. Geriatric patients undergoing appendectomy have increased risk of intraoperative perforation and/or abscess. Surgery. 2020;**168**(2):322-328. DOI: 10.1016/j.surg.2020.04.013

[45] Siddharthan RV, Byrne RM, Dewey E, et al. Appendiceal cancer masked as inflammatory appendicitis in the elderly: Not an uncommon presentation. Journal of Surgical Oncology. 2019;**120**(6):736-740. DOI: 10.1002/jso.25549

[46] Flum DR, Koepsell T, Heagerty P, et al. Appendicitis in patients with acquired immunodeficiency syndrome. Journal of the American College of Surgeons. 1997;**184**(5):481-486. DOI: 10.1016/S1072-7515(97)00162-6

[47] Nguyen A, Lotfollahzadeh S. Appendectomy. In: StatPearls [Internet]. Treasure Island (FL): StatPearls Publishing; 2024. Available from: https://www.ncbi.nlm.nih.gov/books/NBK580514/

[48] Fischer JE, Raskin KA. Management of acute appendicitis. In: Fischer JE, Brunicardi FC, editors. Surgery: Basic Science and Clinical Evidence. 8th ed. New York: McGraw-Hill; 2022. pp. 123-130

[49] Margenthaler JA, Longo WE, Virgo KS, et al. Risk factors for adverse outcomes after the surgical treatment of appendicitis in adults. Annals of Surgery. 2003;**238**(1):59-66. DOI: 10.1097/01.SLA.0000074961.50020.f8

[50] Ferzli GS, Fingerhut A. Trocar placement for laparoscopic abdominal procedures: A simple standardized method. Journal of the American College of Surgeons. 2004;**198**(1):163-173. DOI: 10.1016/j.jamcollsurg.2003.08.031

[51] Veziant J, Slim K. Laparoscopic appendectomy. Journal of Visceral Surgery. 2014;**151**(3):223-228. DOI: 10.1016/j.jviscsurg.2014.07.003

[52] Humes DJ, Simpson J. Acute appendicitis. BMJ. 2006;**333**(7567):530-534. DOI: 10.1136/bmj.38940.664363.AE

[53] Arang H, El Boghdady M. Robotic appendicectomy: A review of feasibility. Sultan Qaboos University Medical Journal. 2023;**23**(4):440-446. DOI: 10.18295/squmj.7.2023.043

[54] Becker T, DeLeon G, Rao V, Pei KY. A comparison of outcomes between laparoscopic and robotic appendectomy among ACS-NSQIP hospitals. Laparoscopic, Endoscopic and Robotic Surgery. 2023;**6**(2):39-42. DOI: 10.1016/j.lers.2023.04.003

[55] Coletta D, Patriti A. Robotic appendectomy. In: Scrub Nurse in Minimally Invasive and Robotic General

Surgery. Cham: Springer International Publishing; 2024. pp. 133-138

[56] St Peter SD, Adibe OO, Juang D, et al. Single incision versus standard 3-port laparoscopic appendectomy: A prospective randomized trial. Annals of Surgery. 2011;**254**(4):586-590. DOI: 10.1097/SLA.0b013e31822b8e5d

[57] Sohn M, Hess S, Boese CK, et al. Surgical management of acute appendicitis in adults: A review of current techniques. International Journal of Surgery. 2017;**48**:232-239. DOI: 10.1016/j.ijsu.2017.11.028

[58] Wei B, Qi CL, Chen TF, et al. Laparoscopic versus open appendectomy for acute appendicitis: A metaanalysis. Surgical Endoscopy. 2011;**25**(4):1199-1208. DOI: 10.1007/s00464-010-1344-z

[59] Biondi A, Di Stefano C, Ferrara F, et al. Laparoscopic versus open appendectomy: A retrospective cohort study assessing outcomes and cost-effectiveness. World Journal of Emergency Surgery: WJES. 2016;**11**(1):44. DOI: 10.1186/s13017-016-0102-5

[60] Stryja J. Surgical site infection and local management of the wound: A meta-analysis. Rozhledy v Chirurgii. 2021;**100**(7):313-324. DOI: 10.48095/rozhlchir2021133

[61] Danwang C, Bigna JJ, Tochie JN, et al. Global incidence of surgical site infection after appendectomy: A systematic review and meta-analysis. BMJ Open. 2020;**10**(2):e034266. DOI: 10.1136/bmjopen-2019-034266

[62] Bhangu A, Søreide K, Di Saverio S, et al. Acute appendicitis: Modern understanding of pathogenesis, diagnosis, and management. Lancet. 2015;**386**(10000):1278-1287. DOI: 10.1016/S0140-6736(15)00275-5

[63] Krisher SL, Browne A, Dibbins A, Tkacz N, Curci M. Intra-abdominal abscess after laparoscopic appendectomy for perforated appendicitis. Archives of Surgery. 2001;**136**(4):438-441. DOI: 10.1001/archsurg.136.4.438

[64] Mulita F, Plachouri KM, Liolis E, Kehagias D, Kehagias I. Comparison of intra-abdominal abscess formation after laparoscopic and open appendectomy for complicated and uncomplicated appendicitis: A retrospective study. Wideochir Inne Tech Maloinwazyjne. 2021;**16**(3):560-565. DOI: 10.5114/wiitm.2021.103942

[65] Kumar A, Sharma A, Khullar R, Soni V, Baijal M, Chowbey PK. Stump appendicitis: A rare clinical entity. Journal of Minimal Access Surgery. 2013;**9**(4):173-176. DOI: 10.4103/0972-9941.118835

[66] Kanona H, Al Samaraee A, Nice C, Bhattacharya V. Stump appendicitis: A review. International Journal of Surgery. 2012;**10**(9):425-428. DOI: 10.1016/j.ijsu.2012.08.016

[67] Dimaya RM, Sahu N. Stump appendicitis. International Journal of Surgery. 2020;**7**(7):2461-2463. DOI: 10.18203/2349-2902.ISJ20202872

[68] Agostinho N, Bains HK, Sardelic F. Enterocutaneous fistula secondary to stump appendicitis. Case Reports in Surgery. 2017;**2017**:6135251. DOI: 10.1155/2017/6135251

[69] Choi PW. Incarcerated incisional hernia of the sigmoid colon after appendectomy: A case report. International Journal of Surgery Case

Reports. 2017;**31**:39-42. DOI: 10.1016/j.ijscr.2017.01.006

[70] Hamouda Ehab SM, Tan BC, Peh WC. Interstitial incisional hernia following appendectomy. Singapore Medical Journal. 2013;**54**(9):531-532. DOI: 10.11622/smedj.2013177

Chapter 4

Minimally Invasive Approach of Appendicular Abscesses in Complicated Acute Appendicitis

José Sebastião dos Santos, Ricardo Ribeiro Correa Filho, Jorge Elias Junior, Rafael Kemp, Ajith Kumar Sankarankutty, Leonardo Resende Sousa and Marcos Antônio Marton Filho

Abstract

Acute appendicitis, complicated by free or blocked perforation with phlegmon and appendiceal abscess, is associated with increased morbidity and mortality, which is less than 0.1% in the non-gangrenous form and reaches approximately 5% in the perforated form. Initial treatment of appendiceal mass with abscess can be performed with antibiotic therapy and a minimally invasive approach. Age, sex, and findings from the history, physical examination, and imaging evaluation support decision-making and guide the use of the most frequently used access routes: percutaneous, transrectal, and transvaginal. Information on technical advances and results, emphasizing resolution time and the need for reapproach, should be further studied to define the level of evidence for the minimally invasive approach in appendiceal abscess.

Keywords: appendicitis, appendiceal abscess, non-operative management, percutaneous drainage, ultrasound-guided drainage, transvaginal drainage, transrectal drainage

1. Introduction

The diagnosis and treatment of acute appendicitis are still challenging, despite its high prevalence. Classification between uncomplicated and complicated appendicitis is essential for selecting treatment.

In uncomplicated appendicitis, the organ is inflamed without signs of gangrene, perforation, intraperitoneal purulent fluid, contained phlegmon, or intra-abdominal abscess [1]. The non-complicated forms are usually treated by appendicectomy (**Figure 1**).

Complicated appendicitis is characterized by gangrene of the inflamed organ with or without perforation, intra-abdominal abscess, contained peri-appendiceal phlegmon, or purulent free fluid [1]. It affects 17–32% of patients [2] and may lead to peritonitis, bowel obstruction, and sepsis.

IntechOpen

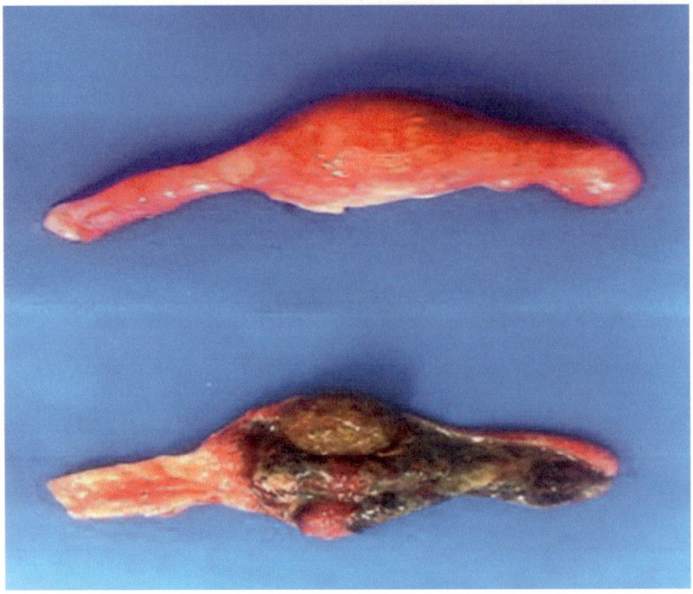

Figure 1.
Cecal appendix without complications with the presence of the appendicolith inside and the obstruction effects (appendix content stasis plus the mucus that continues to be produced, which causes mucosal ischemia and necrosis). The appendicectomy realized at the appropriate timing prevents necrosis in all the layers and the free or blocked perforation of the organ.

Delayed diagnosis or intervention are independent risk factors for perforation [2, 3]. However, it is still debated whether prolonged delay in pre-admission of patients is associated with an increased rate of perforation because there are epidemiological, immunological, and pathological data supporting that acute appendicitis is not a progressive disease, but there are two types of appendicitis: uncomplicated and complicated [4, 5].

On the other hand, the difficulties of primary care teams in making the etiological diagnosis plus the prescription of symptomatic medications and antibiotics, as well as the limit of timely access to hospital reference services in health systems with access ordered by medical regulation [6], are present in the condition illustrated in **Figure 2**.

The imaging findings (**Figure 2**) and adverse events of extensive surgical intervention in appendiceal phlegmon are the outcomes represented in the case of a 70-year-old patient admitted with abdominal pain and diarrhea for 15 days, initially treated for urinary infection in a primary and medium-complexity service.

After a discreet recovery, she was referred to a tertiary hospital, conscious, oriented, and dehydrated, with a heart rate of 96 beats per minute and a respiratory rate of 36 incursions per minute, an arterial blood pressure of 176/97 mmHg, and an oxygen saturation of 91%. There was a palpable and painful mass in the right hemiabdomen, with a defensive reaction in the site. Complementary exams: Hemoglobin 10.7 (reference value of 15.0 ± 2.0 g/dL); white blood cell: 15.300 (reference value of 4.000–10.000/mm^3); rod cells: 17 (reference value of 4–5%); platelet: 765 (reference value of 150–400 × 109/L); creatinine: 0.89 (reference value of 0.50–1.20 mg/dL); glycemia: 123 (reference value of 70–99 mg/dL); C-reactive protein: 1.93 (reference value lower than 0.3 mg/dL); and lactate of 1.7 (reference value of 0.63–2.44 mmol/L). In addition to the systemic alterations correction measures, plus antibiotic therapy, there was an improvement in the heart rate to 78 beats per minute and respiratory rate to 18 incursions per minute with an oxygen saturation of 95%.

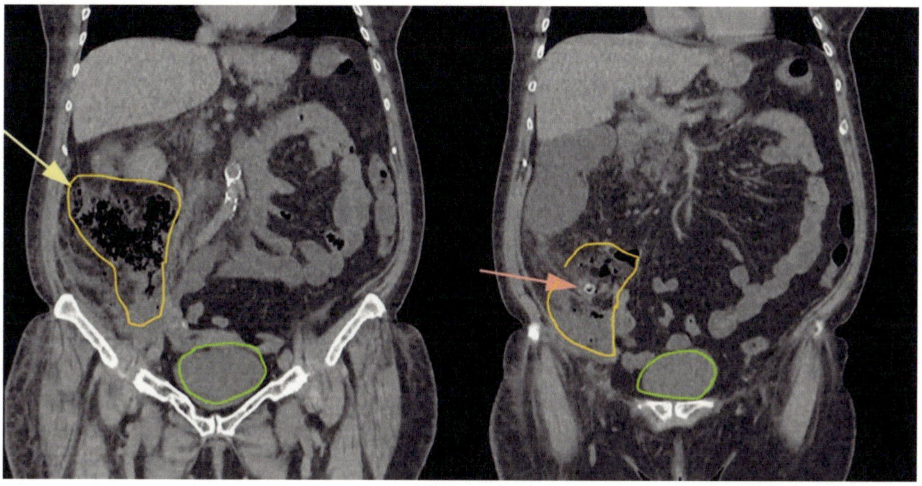

Figure 2.
Computed tomography scan showing a localized abscess (yellow arrow) with an associated appendicolith (red arrow) and the bladder highlighted in green.

The percutaneous drainage proceeded, showing an exit of fecaloid secretion, and an exploratory laparotomy was indicated. A right colectomy was performed with side-to-side anastomosis between the ileum and transverse colon, and the abdomen was left in peritoneostomy. During the postoperative period, the patient required invasive respiratory support, low dosages of vasoactive drugs, evolving with kidney failure, requiring hemodialysis, embolism of low charge, worsening of hemodynamic instability, and exit of enteric secretion through the draining tube. The patient was reoperated with identification of dehiscence of the transversal ilium anastomosis and evolved with sepsis, multiple organ insufficiency, and death, 38 days after admission.

In the circumstances described, the blocked form was present at the time of diagnosis with appendiceal abscess, and the surgical approach is associated with extensive resections (ileotyphlectomy or right colectomy). The rate of ileocecal resection in emergency appendectomy is very high (50%) when compared to interval appendectomy, performed between 8 and 12 weeks (3%), as are the rates of postoperative complications, respectively, 75% and 9% [7].

The lesson learned is that antibiotic therapy and a minimally invasive approach may be used to treat the initial appendiceal mass with abscess or delimited phlegmon. Age, gender, history findings, physical exams, and image evaluation guide decision-making and the use of different access routes: percutaneous, transrectal, and transvaginal. Information about technological advances and results for a minimally invasive approach in appendiceal abscess, focusing on timing resolution and re-approaching requirements, must be further studied to better define evidence.

Elderly patients are more likely than other age groups to have appendicitis complicated by perforation or abscess. The rate of complicated appendicitis ranges from 18% to 70% (compared with a rate ranging from 3% to 29% among patients younger than 65 years of age) [8, 9]. The mortality is significantly higher in elderly patients with perforated appendicitis compared to elderly patients with non-perforated ones (15% vs. 3%) [10, 11].

2. Clinical presentation and complicated appendicitis diagnosis

Patients admitted with blocked forms of acute appendicitis show an atypical evolution with an extended history and may represent an additional challenge for diagnosis. Despite the disease's clinical predictors, the presence of a palpable mass in the right iliac fossa or unspecific painful conditions are indications of a complementary exam requirement, above all ultrasound and tomography.

The symptoms duration, the clinical impact, the systemic involvement, the laboratory exam disorders, and the image findings frequently identified in complicated appendicitis cases are relevant to the decision-making.

Among the forms of complicated acute appendicitis presentation, the characterization of the clinical and image presentation is essential [12]:

- Phlegmon: inflammatory mass of softened tissue around the appendix.
- Periappendicular abscess: collection with peripherical wall increased on computerized tomography, with intravenous contrast or peripheral hyperemic ring with color Doppler on ultrasonography.
- Highlighted defects on the appendiceal wall.
- Extraluminal air.
- Extraluminal appendicoliths.

3. Drainage routes of periappendicular abscess

The non-surgical approach for appendicitis described in 1901 [13] is the best therapeutic alternative for the blocked forms of complicated acute appendicitis, exactly because it reduces complications associated with extended resections, surgical manipulation with loss of anatomical references, and increases morbidity and lethality [13].

Antibiotic treatment must be immediately instituted, and the choice must contemplate covers for anaerobic and gram-negative germs. There are pieces of evidence for the use of penicillins associated with beta-lactamase inhibitors (clavulin), in addition to cephalosporins and quinolones associated with metronidazole [14].

The abscess drainage guided by image is indicated also at an early stage, guided by ultrasonography (US) or computerized tomography (CT) to treat the local inflammation. The procedure is realized under local anesthesia and shows a low rate of complications [15].

Patients with good clinical progress may be submitted to surgical treatment after 6–12 weeks from drainage (interval appendectomy), due to the recurrence risk of the disease. However, this interval for surgery needs robust evidence and is indicated only with histopathological aspects of inflammation [7, 16]. A new image exam must document the abscess resolution before removing the drain tube and dismissing the patient from the hospital.

The risk of recurrence of appendicitis with abscess after conservative treatment ranges from 7% to 24% [17, 18]. The interval appendectomy after drainage of appendiceal abscesses should not be performed routinely. At the same time, patients with risk factors may require additional investigation to exclude secondary diagnoses of appendiceal abscesses, such as neoplasms and Crohn's disease, requiring additional investigation with performing a colonoscopy.

The preoperative colonoscopy execution to study appendicitis etiology is indicated for adult patients due to the possibility of neoplasias in the population aged 40 years or older who are at higher risk of exhibiting malignant, and eventually, Crohn's disease (**Figure 3**) [7, 19].

Interval appendicectomy—two arms elective surgery and follow-up observation only.

On the other hand, there is a randomized clinical trial demonstrating that emergency laparoscopic appendectomy is a viable and safe first-line treatment option for appendicitis with abscess when performed by experienced surgeons. In this study, emergency laparoscopic treatment had a lower readmission rate (3% vs. 27%) and a lower rate of additional intervention (7% vs. 30%) compared to conservative treatment. Conversion to laparotomy was necessary in 10% of patients who underwent laparoscopic treatment and in 13% of patients who received conservative treatment [20].

Patients with intra-abdominal collection associated with generalized peritonitis, hemodynamic instability, and clinical signs of sepsis must be submitted to laparotomy or laparoscopy right after the initial stabilization. Multiple abscesses, not communicating, with associated fistulas must also be treated with surgical drainage. The single collection, or in a lower number, communicating, are eligible for minimally invasive drainage [16].

Age, gender, and physical constitution, in addition to the collection location, must be factors considered for decision-making regarding the best access route for draining the abscess.

3.1 Percutaneous drainage

Pelvic abscess placed above the line formed by the femoral heads, in addition to the ones in the abdominal topography, allows percutaneous drainage guided by US [20–24]. Collections placed inside the abdominal wall, Retzius space (pre-vesicular), superior, anterior, or anterolateral to the bladder are also benefited from the percutaneous drainage [16].

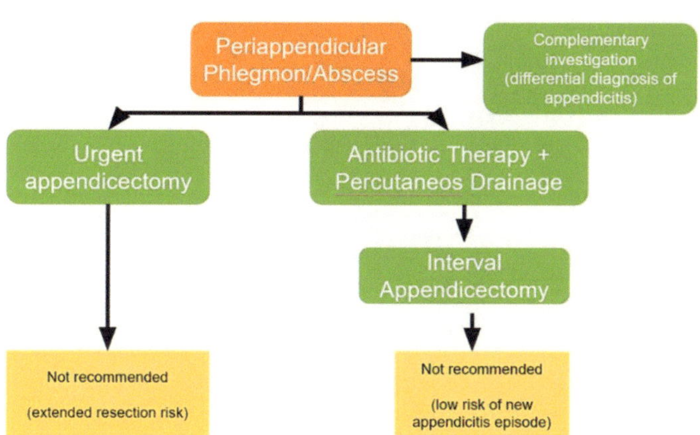

Figure 3.
Suggested algorithm for management of periappendiceal phlegmon/abscess and interval appendectomy.

3.2 Transrectal drainage

Transrectal drainage of pelvic abscesses is well established in children and courses with high rates of resolution after the procedure [25].

More recently, the transrectal approach is also used for the treatment of deep pelvic abscesses in adult patients, especially in male patients.

Collection on the rectovesical spaces, presacral, between the sacral and the rectum, and perirectal show a high rate of resolution after transrectal drainage guided by US [16]. The sequence of images in **Figure 4** shows the evolution of a patient submitted to abscess draining guided by the transrectal US, with collection reduction on the control tomography 6 days past the draining.

The male patient was 26 years old and had abdominal pain in the hypogastric region for 7 days, associated with nausea and vomiting, hyporexia, and progressed to aqueous diarrhea and fever. Physical finding: feverish, defense and pain to superficial and deep palpation, and abrupt decompression on the right iliac fossa and suprapubic region. Complementary exam findings: increase of the C-reactive protein: 12.99 (reference value lower than 0.3 mg/dL) and of the lactate of 2.6 (reference value of 0.63–2.44 mmol/L). The patient was treated with amoxicillin and clavulanic acid for 10 days and submitted to a transrectal echoendoscopy, puncture, and emptying of three stores. He's been asymptomatic for 8 years.

3.3 Transvaginal drainage

The transvaginal approach has been gaining space with the improvement of image exam techniques for the treatment of collection in female patients. The collections located adjacent to the deep uterine, vesicouterine spaces, and recto-uterine spaces (Pouch of Douglas) are favorable for transvaginal drainage guided by the US [16].

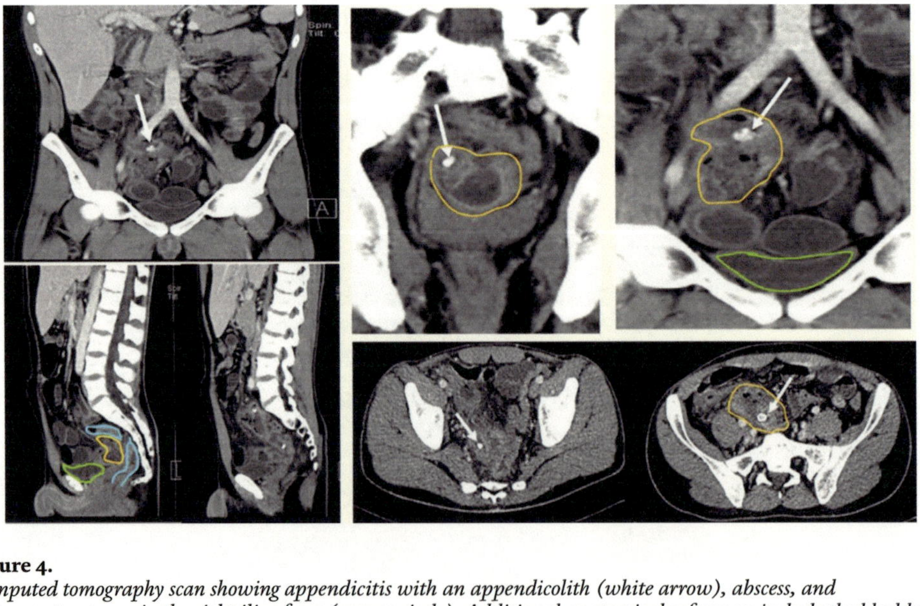

Figure 4.
Computed tomography scan showing appendicitis with an appendicolith (white arrow), abscess, and inflammatory mass in the right iliac fossa (orange circle). Additional anatomical references include the bladder (green circle) and rectum (blue circle).

4. Final considerations

- The clinical presentations dragged or with a mass on the right iliac fossa indicate the necessity of complementary diagnoses with images.
- Patients with clinical signs of peritonitis, hemodynamic instability, or sepsis are not eligible for minimally invasive approaches and must be submitted to laparotomy or laparoscopy.
- Blocked complicated acute appendicitis (for phlegmon or abscess) must be treated, preferably through a minimally invasive route and antibiotic therapy.
- Clinical and imaging characteristics of the collections must be considered for a minimally invasive approach.
- The choice of the access route (percutaneous, transrectal, or transvaginal) depends on the location as determined by images of the pelvic/abdominal collection (**Figure 5**).

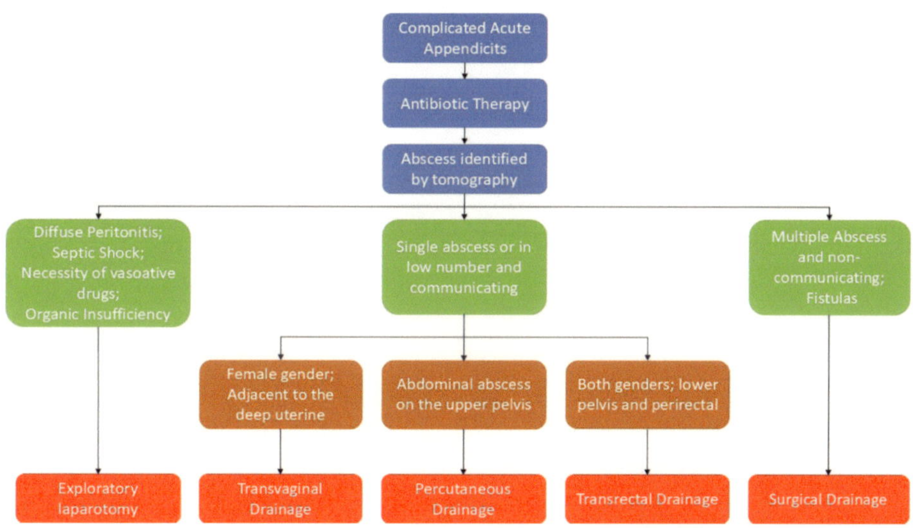

Figure 5.
Suggest algorithm for approaching the periappendiceal abscess on complicated acute appendicitis.

Author details

José Sebastião dos Santos[1*], Ricardo Ribeiro Correa Filho[2], Jorge Elias Junior[1], Rafael Kemp[1], Ajith Kumar Sankarankutty[1], Leonardo Resende Sousa[2] and Marcos Antônio Marton Filho[3]

1 Ribeirão Preto Medical School, University of São Paulo, Ribeirão Preto, Brasil

2 Clinical Hospital of the Faculty of Medicine of Ribeirão Preto of the University of São Paulo, Ribeirão Preto, Brasil

3 Bauru Medical School, University of São Paulo, Bauru, Brasil

*Address all correspondence to: jsdsanto@fmrp.usp.br

IntechOpen

© 2025 The Author(s). Licensee IntechOpen. This chapter is distributed under the terms of the Creative Commons Attribution License (http://creativecommons.org/licenses/by/4.0), which permits unrestricted use, distribution, and reproduction in any medium, provided the original work is properly cited.

References

[1] Ramon RG, Hasan HE, Marguerite AW, et al. Diagnosis and management of acute appendicitis. EAES consensus development conference 2015. Surgical Endoscopy. 2016;**30**:4668-4690. DOI: 10.1007/s00464-016-5245-7

[2] Mandeville K, Monuteaux M, Pottker T, Bulloch B. Effects of timing to diagnosis and appendectomy in pediatric appendicitis. Pediatric Emergency Care. 2015;**31**(11):753-758. DOI: 10.1097/PEC.0000000000000596

[3] Snyder MJ, Guthrie M, Cagle S. Acute appendicitis: Efficient diagnosis and management. American Family Physician. 2018;**98**(1):25-33

[4] Barreto SG, Travers E, Thomas T, et al. Acute perforated appendicitis: An analysis of risk factors to guide surgical decision making. Indian Journal of Medical Sciences. 2010;**64**(2):58-65. DOI: 10.4103/0019-5359.94401

[5] Andersson RE. The natural history and traditional management of appendicitis revisited: Spontaneous resolution and predominance of prehospital perforations imply that a correct diagnosis is more important than an early diagnosis. World Journal of Surgery. 2007;**31**:86-92

[6] Lopes SLB, dos Santos JS, Scarpelini S. The implementation of the Medical Regulation Office and Mobile Emergency Attendance System and its impact on the gravity profile of non-traumatic afflictions treated in a University Hospital: A research study. BMC Health Services Research. 2007;7:173. DOI: 10.1186/1472-6963-7-173

[7] Suzuki T, Matsumoto A, Akao T, Matsumoto H. Interval appendectomy as a safe and feasible treatment after conservative treatment for appendicitis with abscess: A retrospective, single-center cohort study. Updates in Surgery. 2023;**75**(8):2257-2265. DOI: 10.1007/s13304-023-01679-1

[8] Kraemer M, Franke C, Ohmann C, et al. Acute appendicitis in late adulthood: Incidence, presentation, and outcome. Results of a prospective multicenter acute abdominal pain study and a review of the literature. Langenbeck's Archives of Surgery. 2000;**385**(7):470-481

[9] Fugazzola P, Ceresoli M, Agnoletti V, et al. The SIFIPAC/WSES/SICG/SIMEU guidelines for diagnosis and treatment of acute appendicitis in the elderly (2019 edition). World Journal of Emergency Surgery : WJES. 2020;**15**(1):19. DOI: 10.1186/s13017-020-00298-0

[10] Gürleyik G, Gürleyik E. Age-related clinical features in older patients with acute appendicitis. European Journal of Emergency Medicine. 2003;**10**(3):200-203. DOI: 10.1097/00063110-200309000-00008

[11] Lunca S, Bouras G, Romedea NS. Acute appendicitis in the elderly patient: Diagnostic problems, prognostic factors and outcomes. Romanian Journal of Gastroenterology. 2004;**13**(4):299-303

[12] Borruel Nacenta S, Ibáñez Sanz L, Sanz LR, et al. Update on acute appendicitis: Typical and untypical findings. Radiología (English Edition). 2023;**65**(Suppl. 1):S81-S91. DOI: 10.1016/j.rxeng.2022.09.010

[13] Ochsnerv AJ. The cause of diffuse peritonitis complicating appendicitis and

its prevention. Journal of the American Medical Association. 1901;**26**:1747-1754

[14] Sallinen V, Akl EA, You JJ, et al. Meta-analysis of antibiotics versus appendicectomy for non-perforated acute appendicitis. The British Journal of Surgery. 2016;**103**(6):656-667

[15] Sudakoff GS, Lundeen SJ, Otterson MF. Transrectal and transvaginal sonographic intervention of infected pelvic fluid collections: A complete approach. Ultrasound Quarterly. 2005;**21**(3):175-185. DOI: 10.1097/01.ruq.0000174753.16708.7a

[16] Demetrashvili Z, Kenchadze G, Pipia I, et al. Comparison of treatment methods of appendiceal mass and abscess: A prospective cohort study. Annals of Medicine and Surgery. 2019;**48**:48-52. DOI: 10.1016/j.amsu.2019.10.016

[17] Renteria O, Shahid Z, Huerta S. Outcomes of appendectomy in elderly veteran patients. Surgery. 2018;**164**:460-465. DOI: 10.1016/j.surg.2018.04.02

[18] Tingstedt B, Bexe-Lindskog E, Ekelund M, Andersson R. Management of appendiceal masses. The European Journal of Surgery. 2002;**168**:579-582

[19] Corfield L. Interval appendectomy after appendiceal mass or abscess in adults: What is "best practice"? Surgery Today. 2007;**37**:1-4. DOI: 10.1007/s00595-006-3334-2

[20] Mentula P, Sammalkorpi H, Leppäniemi A. Laparoscopic surgery or conservative treatment for appendiceal abscess in adults? A randomized controlled trial. Annals of Surgery. 2015, 2015;**262**:237-242. DOI: 10.1097/SLA.0000000000001200

[21] Lai HW, Loong CC, Chiu JH, Chau GY, Wu CW, Lui WY. Interval appendectomy after conservative treatment of an appendiceal mass. World Journal of Surgery. Mar 2006;**30**(3):352-357. DOI: 10.1007/s00268-005-0128-4

[22] American College of Radiology. Percutaneous catheter drainage of infected intra-abdominal fluid collections. In: ACR Appropriateness Criteria. Reston, VA: American College of Radiology; 1999

[23] Gazelle GS, Mueller PR. Abdominal abscesses: Imaging and intervention. Radiologic Clinics of North America. 1994;**32**:913-932

[24] VanSonnenberg E, Ferrucci JT, Mueller PR, et al. Percutaneous drainage of abscesses and fluid collections: Technique, results, and applications. Radiology. 1982;**142**:1-10

[25] McDaniel JD, Warren MT, Pence JC, Ey EH. Ultrasound-guided transrectal drainage of deep pelvic abscesses in children: A modified and simplified technique. Pediatric Radiology. 2015;**45**(3):435-438. DOI: 10.1007/s00247-014-3154-2. Epub 2014 Sep 14

Section 2

Pediatric Appendicitis

Chapter 5

Diagnosing Acute Appendicitis in Children: The Role of Diagnostic Scores

Adelais K. Tzortzopoulou

Abstract

Appendicitis is one of the most common emergency conditions in children. Through inflammation, necrosis, and perforation of the appendix layers, it causes often peritonitis. Recent epidemiological and clinical data support the theory of two distinct pathological entities of appendicitis: simple non-perforated and complicated appendicitis. Simple non-perforated appendicitis in children can be treated successfully with antibiotics in 92% of cases; thus, complicated appendicitis proceeds rapidly to perforation and should be managed with emergency surgery. To approach acute appendicitis, a lot of clinical scoring systems have been created, which are easily applicable to pediatric patients and their parents due to their simple variables consisting of clinical symptoms, physical examination findings, and laboratory data. Clinical score systems (as PAS and Alvarado Score) currently in practice cannot predict which children with appendicitis should proceed directly to surgery. As a result, preoperative ultrasound (US) and/or low-dose CT scan imaging is recommended in all intermediate or high-risk patients in order to diagnose them properly. CoApPS score is a recently presented score that could guide doctors, both experienced and inexperienced ones in emergency management of children with complicated appendicitis reducing hospitalizations and urgent surgeries. A combination of positive jumping-up test, vomiting, White Blood Cell count >13.5 x 10^{-3}/ml, lymphocytes <18% and C-reactive protein >50 mg/dl are the score's predictors. In this chapter, we will discuss the scores that are nowadays used to diagnose appendicitis in children, focusing on the advantages and disadvantages of each scoring system, and comparing them with each other.

Keywords: appendicitis, children, diagnostic scores, PAS, Alvarado score, CoApP score

1. Introduction

Acute appendicitis is one of the most common emergency conditions in children. Annually, more than 250,000 new cases are reported worldwide. It still remains a diagnostic dilemma for clinicians because the symptoms and signs are not specific, mimicking a pleiad of pathology, such as gastroenteritis, mesenteric lymphadenitis, Meckel's diverticulitis, torsion of intraabdominal organs, etc. The diagnosis commonly demands surgical consultation, a hospital stay, and sometimes

IntechOpen

advanced CT imaging studies when the clinical examination and the ultrasound are not pathognomonic for the disease. Misdiagnosis can lead to an increased rate of complications and critical conditions, such as perforation and peritonitis, intraabdominal abscess, and sepsis [1].

To approach acute appendicitis, a lot of clinical score systems have been created, which are easily applicable to pediatric patients and their parents, due to their simple variables consisting of clinical symptoms, physical examination findings, and laboratory data. Alvarado in 1986 with a focus on identifying patients with abdominal pain requiring surgery presented the first acute appendicitis score in adults with a sensitivity of 81% and a specificity of 74%. In 2002 Samuel introduced the first appendicitis scoring system specifically for children, the Pediatric Appendicitis Score (PAS). This score consists of six clinical and two laboratory parameters. 8 years later in 2010, the RIPASA score was introduced to diagnose acute appendicitis in Asian patients. Later, other scoring systems were proposed, such as the Appendicitis Inflammatory Score (AIR), the Adult Appendicitis Score (AAS), and the Sonographic Score, an ultrasound scale for evaluating the inflamed appendix. In addition, the Heidelberg Acute Appendicitis (HAS) score for children was proposed in 2017, which is also based on a combination of clinical symptoms, laboratory and ultrasound findings. In the last 20 years, numerous studies have been carried out in children, studying these scores, their reliability in diagnosing the disease, but also their ability to minimize the frequency of negative appendectomies and false-negative cases with failure to diagnose the disease (missed cases), increasing complications [2–5].

It is also very important to mention that for centuries it was thought that appendicitis was a progressive disease-causing peritonitis through inflammation, necrosis, and perforation of appendix layers. Recent epidemiological and clinical data strongly support the concept of two different types of appendicitis with different cause and prognosis: simple non-perforated appendicitis and complicated appendicitis. Complicated appendicitis proceeds rapidly to perforation and should be managed with emergency surgery in children. On the other hand, simple appendicitis can be treated successfully with antibiotics in 92% of cases. Clinical score systems currently in practice have the potential to correctly stratify these children who could be considered for early discharge as low-risk patients. Unfortunately, they cannot predict which children with appendicitis should proceed directly to surgery. That was the reason that the last 5 years the whole pediatric community is searching for new scores to distinguish one entity from the other in simple ways, in order to minimize the complications and to choose the most suitable therapy for each patient [6].

In the next pages we will first discuss about all the scores are nowadays used to diagnose appendicitis in children, focusing on the advantages and disadvantages of each scoring system, comparing them with each other. We will also discuss about the newest scores which are specifically used for diagnosing complicated appendicitis and the usefulness of the previous ones in distinguishing simple appendicitis from complicated.

2. Alvarado score

The Alvarado scoring system includes clinical symptoms and signs as well as simple laboratory blood tests, which form the code MANTRELS. This score consists of eight prognostic factors, each of which is scored with 1 or 2 points (**Table 1**).

	Alvarado scoring system	PAS
Symptoms		
Migration of pain	1	1
Anorexia	1	1
Nausea and/or Vomiting	1	1
Signs Right lower quadrant tenderness		
Rebound pain	1	2
Temperature > 37.3°C	1	-
Temperature > 38°C	-	1
Laboratory		
Leukocytosis > 10 x 10^3	2	1
Polymorphonuclear neutrophilia (NE) >75%	1	1
Total	10	10

Source: Refs. [2, 5].

Table 1.
Alvarado scoring system and pediatric appendicitis score (PAS).

An Alvarado score of less than 5 is considered to rule out the disease with sufficient sensitivity (greater than 95%), but cannot rule in the diagnosis of acute appendicitis in children because it has less specificity of the required (usually greater than 85%). A total score of 5 or 6 suggests appendicitis, but careful patient monitoring, clinical reassessment, and ultrasonography are required. A score of 7 or 8 strengthens the diagnosis of appendicitis, while with a score of 9 or 10, it is almost certain that the patient has acute appendicitis, and surgery is recommended [2, 7].

A meta-analysis of the Alvarado score by Ohle in 2011 in 1635 pediatric patients showed a sensitivity of 99% and a specificity of 57% with a required cut-off score of 5 for admission to a pediatric surgery clinic. These results are equal to those in adult patients, where the score has a sensitivity of 87% and a specificity of 76% with a cut-off of seven. It should be mentioned, that in this meta-analysis the pediatric patient population was heterogeneous regarding age and there is nothing mentioned about the sensitivity and specificity of the score in age subgroups. In 2017 Peyvasteh et al. published results of the Alvarado scale in 400 children under 12 years old with suspected appendicitis. Patients were evaluated with a modified Alvarado scale, which included one more parameter, white shift to left. Sensitivity was 91.3%, specificity 38.4%, positive predictive value 87.7%, and negative predictive value 51.2% [8–10].

Goncalves et al. in a study including 192 children (aged 4–17 years) observed that as the cut-off of the Alvarado scale score decreases, the sensitivity and specificity increase while the positive predictive value and negative predictive value decrease. Equivalent results were reported in a systematic review by Heineman, who concluded that more research is needed so that the Alvarado scale could be used safely without imaging studies in order to diagnose acute appendicitis in children [11, 12].

Table 2 indicatively the diagnostic characteristics of various studies on the Alvarado scale in acute appendicitis in children.

Score	Sensitivity (%)	Specificity (%)	LR + ve	LR-ve	Literature
=4	98.5	26.9	1.34	0.05	Schneider et al. [13]
> = 5	99	0.57	2.30	0.01	Ohle et al. [8]
> = 7	87	76	3.78	0.17	Ohle et al. [8]
> = 7	89	59	2.17	0.18	Pogorelic et al. [14]
> = 7	91.3	38	1.48	0.23	Peyvatech et al. [9]

Table 2.
Diagnostic characteristics in Alvarado score for diagnosing acute appendicitis in children.

3. Pediatric appendicitis score (PAS)

The PAS' scale is the first acute abdominal pain scoring system designed specifically for children with acute abdominal pain suspecting appendicitis. In 2002, Samuel proposed the Pediatric Appendicitis Score, which includes eight parameters, six clinical, and two laboratories with each of them receiving a value of 1 or 2 points, depending on its diagnostic strength (**Table 3**). The cut-off score of 5 showed that only a small percentage of appendicitis cases crossed the scale. However, a sufficient percentage of negative appendectomies was also observed. A score greater than 6 was compatible with an increased likelihood of appendicitis, and scores of 7–10 indicated a very high likelihood of appendicitis. Samuel suggested the PAS scale as a useful diagnostic tool for acute appendicitis in pediatric populations, with a sensitivity of 100%, specificity of 92%, positive predictive value of 96%, and negative predictive value of 99% [5, 15].

The results of the study on the PAS scale were so encouraging that in the last 10 years, many clinical studies have been done using the PAS in pediatric populations. Thus, Bhatt in 2009 presented a study in 246 children aged 4–18 years with his main observation, that using a score of 5 as a cut-off for appendectomy, the number of false positive diagnoses reached 37.6% (negative appendectomies). However, when children with a PAS score of less than 4 remained for follow-up at home, the sensitivity was 97.6% and the negative predictive value was 97.7%. The conclusion of the study was that in patients with a PAS score greater than 8, surgeons could

	Variable	Value
Symptoms	Migration of pain	1
	Anorexia	1
	Nausea/vomiting	1
Signs	Right lower quadrant tenderness	2
	Rebound pain	2
	Elevation of temperature > 38°C	1
Laboratory	Leukocytosis>10 x 10^9/	1
	Polymorphonuclear neutrophilia>75%	1

Table 3.
Pediatric appendicitis score (PAS).

proceed with appendectomy because the specificity was 95.1% and the positive predictive value was 85.2%. However, Bhatt's results indirectly suggest that patients with a PAS score between 5 and 7 will additionally need imaging studies for a more accurate diagnosis [16–18].

Another study by Prada in 275 children under 15 years showed that PAS is useful in the differential diagnosis of appendicitis from cases of nonspecific abdominal pain in children, but suggested the use of CRP as an additional parameter to refine the scale [19].

A review by Dingemann that included eight studies from 2009 to 2012 comparing Alvarado score and PAS came to the conclusion that these two diagnostic scales are not yet the "gold standard" for diagnosing appendicitis in children, although both achieve high specificities (72–98.2%) and sensitivities (76–100%) [16].

Ebel et al. [20] compared the cut-offs of the diagnostic features of the Alvarado and PAS scales and concluded that the Alvarado scale is superior to the PAS scale in diagnosing low-risk patients for appendicitis. The researchers suggested that patients with an Alvarado score less than 4 should not be screened further because they have only a 3% chance of disease when the relative incidence of acute appendicitis takes any value below 60%. On the other hand, the probability of disease increases up to 86% when the Alvarado score is greater than or equal to 7, in which case surgical treatment is recommended [20].

Pogorelic et al. [14] in the study of 311 children with suspected appendicitis showed that both scales could help in the diagnosis of acute appendicitis in children because no significant difference in sensitivity and specificity was found between these scores when the cut-off for appendectomy was at a score of 7. The authors claimed that PAS has 86% sensitivity, 50% specificity, and 90.1% positive predictive value, while Alvarado has 89% sensitivity, 59% specificity, and 93.1% positive predictive value [14].

In 2018, Song et al. compared the modified Alvarado score with the PAS in 142 children under 10 years old. The children were divided into two groups according to their age: group 1 with preschool children (under 5 years old) and group 2 with children between 5 and 10 years old. This study showed that both scales have low diagnostic accuracy in group 1. In this age group, abscesses and perforations of the appendix were more frequent, a finding that strongly suggests that in these very young patients, both scales are not ideal for the diagnosis of appendicitis, mainly due to the atypical clinical symptoms and difficult communication with the child in this age [21].

Table 4 lists the diagnostic characteristics of various studies on the PAS score in children with acute appendicitis.

Score	Sensitivity (%)	Specificity (%)	LR + ve	LR-ve	References
4	95.9	74.2	3.71	0.05	Schneider et al. [13]
5	92.4	57	2.15	0.13	Schneider et al. [13]
> = 6	90.3	47	1.70	0.20	El-Shamy et al. [22]
> = 7	86	50	1.72	0.28	Pogorelic et al.[14]
> = 7	73.5	85.3	5	0.27	Bhatt et al. [23]

Table 4.
Diagnostic features of the PAS scale in children with acute appendicitis.

4. Appendicitis inflammation response (AIR) score

The AIR score is an acute appendicitis risk scoring system and is the first in the literature to include C-reactive protein (CRP) in its clinical and laboratory parameters (**Table 5**) [24, 25].

In the literature, there are several studies in children with suspected appendicitis that compare the AIR scale with other scoring systems. Macco et al. in a retrospective study including 747 children showed that AIR is a better scoring system than Alvarado or PAS for the diagnosis of acute appendicitis even in children under 6 years of age. In high-risk patients, the AIR score had better specificity, positive predictive value, and negative predictive value. Furthermore, in children evaluated with the AIR scale, the rate of negative appendectomies was only 6%, compared to 24% in the Alvarado score and 36% in the PAS score [22].

Another study by El-Shamy involving 278 children under the age of 18 had the same results as the aforementioned study. The sensitivity, specificity, and positive predictive value of the AIR scale were higher than those of Alvarado or PAS. In low-risk patients with the AIR scale, false-negative rates of acute appendicitis of 2.2% were observed, whereas for Alvarado 4% and for PAS 9.7%. The author claimed that the AIR scoring system is the most accurate system for diagnosing acute appendicitis in children [26].

In a recent retrospective study during the years 2009–2012 in patients with suspected appendicitis from 25 hospitals in Sweden, Andersson et al. [24] reported that the AIR score in children aged less than 15 years, with a score of less than 4 achieves a very high sensitivity (99%), while a score greater than 8 has a very high specificity (98%) [24].

	Score
Vomiting	1
RLQ tenderness	1
Rebound tenderness or muscle rigidity	
Light	1
Medium	2
Strong	3
Body temperature >38.5°C	1
Leukocytosis	
10–14.9x 10^9/L	1
>15x 10^9/L	2
Polymorphonuclear leukocytes shift	
70–84%	1
>85%	2
CRP concentration	
10–49 mg/dl	1
>50 mg/dl	2
Total score	12

Table 5.
Appendicitis inflammation response (AIR) score.

Score	Sensitivity (%)	Specificity (%)	LR + ve	LR-ve	References
<=4	95	74	3.67	0.07	Vasiri et al. [27]
<=4	99	26	1.33	0.03	Andersson et al. [24]
> = 9	19.7	98	9.85	0.82	Andersson et al. [24]
> = 9	97.8	84.3	6.23	0.02	El-Shamy et al. [22]

Table 6.
Diagnostic features of the AIR scale in children with acute appendicitis.

Table 6 lists indicatively the diagnostic characteristics of various studies on the AIR scale in children with suspected appendicitis.

5. Critical consideration of the Alvarado, PAS, and AIR scores with Bayes theory

The Alvarado Score, PAS, and AIR score for children are primarily intended to classify patients into three risk categories: (1) high-risk appendicitis patients, (2) low-risk patients, and (3) intermediate-risk patients. With this classification, it is intended that high-risk patients are admitted to a pediatric surgery clinic for evaluation by specialists and possible surgical treatment, while low-risk patients are monitored for 24 hours, preferably at home. Intermediate-risk patients usually undergo diagnostic imaging to confirm the diagnosis.

From the review of the literature, we found that most authors in their studies on children with the Alvarado, PAS, and AIR scales classify patients into risk groups, having as classification criteria mainly sensitivity, specificity, positive predictive value, and negative predictive value of scales. It should be emphasized, however, that both the positive and negative prognostic value of a risk scale, but also of any diagnostic test, depends on the relative frequency (abusedly understood as "prevalence") of the disease in the sample of the respective population that is being investigated. Therefore, it is considered necessary to use as indicators those diagnostic characteristics, which are completely independent of the relative frequency of the disease in the studied sample of the population. The positive and negative likelihood ratios of the disease (positive Likelihood Ratio, negative Likelihood Ratio) are considered ideal diagnostic characteristics. These characteristics of a scale are the most suitable indicators, on the one hand, for the classification of patients into risk categories and, on the other hand, for the comparative evaluation of the various scales that are applied to children's populations with a different relative frequency of acute appendicitis each time [28–31].

With the probability quotients achieved by each scale and with the relative frequency of the disease in each population, we can calculate the % post-test probability of disease of the patients, so that they can be classified based on the post-test probability - probabilities for each risk group (Bayes theory). In this way, as high risk for appendicitis, we can conventionally consider patients with a post-test probability greater than 85%, low-risk patients with a post-test probability of less than 1%, and intermediate-risk all the rest.

Table 7 compares the meta-probabilities of acute appendicitis in Alvarado, PAS, and AIR scores, as we calculated them based on odds ratios in pediatric populations with different frequencies of the disease.

SCORE	Meta-probabilities of acute appedicitis						LR	References
Alvarado<5	2.91	1.99	1.31	*0.85*	0.50	0.22	0.02	Schneider et al. [13]
Alvarado > = 7	79.17	79.16	71.69	61.96	48.71	29.69	3.8	Ohle et al. [8]
PAS <5	6.98	4.76	3.22	2.09	*1.23*	0.55	0.05	Schneider et al. [13]
PAS > =7	83.33	83.33	76.92	51.72	55.55	35.71	5	Bhatt et al. [23]
AIR<5	4.3	2.91	1.96	*1.26*	0.74	0.33	0.03	Andersson et al. [24]
AIR > = 9	93.66	90.77	*86.78*	80.87	71.11	52.25	9.85	Andersson et al. [24]
AIR > = 9 (complicated appendicitis)	96.05	94.18	91.54	*87.44*	80.24	64.36	16.25	Andersson et al. [24]
Frequency (%) of acute appendicitis	*60*	*50*	*40*	*30*	*20*	*10*		

Table 7.
Meta-probabilities of acute appendicitis in Alvarado, PAS and AIR scores in pediatric populations with different frequency of the disease.

From the information listed in **Table 7**, it follows that the Alvarado scale with a score below 5 presents the smallest negative probability quotient (LR-ve = 0.02) of the other two scales, but cannot rule out the disease with a post probability of appendicitis below 1%, except in populations with a relative incidence of disease below 40%. It is also clear that the Alvarado scale with LR + ve 3.8 fails to diagnose acute appendicitis in patients with a scale score greater than or equal to 7 in any of the populations with a relative incidence of disease equal to or less than 60%, because the odds of disease with this scale they remain smaller than the required limit of 85% [8, 16].

On the PAS scale patients with a score below 5 have a probability of acute appendicitis below 1%, but only if they belong to populations with a relative incidence of disease below 20%, in which case these patients will be able to remain for follow-up at home. Patients with a PAS score equal to or greater than 7 do not approach the threshold for disease diagnosis (probability greater than 85%), except in populations with a relative incidence of disease greater than 50%. Therefore, the PAS scale can exclude the diagnosis only in populations with a low relative frequency of appendicitis, while it approaches the critical limit of diagnosis exclusively in populations with a very high relative frequency of the disease [13, 32].

An AIR score of less than 5 cannot rule out acute appendicitis in children except in populations with a relative disease incidence of less than 30%. At the same time, it presents the possibility of diagnosing the disease in general with a score greater than or equal to 9, but only in populations with a relative frequency of appendicitis greater than 30%. The ability to diagnose complicated appendicitis with the AIR scale also concerns mainly populations with a relative incidence of disease equal to or greater than 30% [13].

6. Scoring systems including imaging techniques

Many pediatric hospitals in order to improve the diagnosis of appendicitis are using imaging protocols together with imaging scoring systems. In the US scan

1	Completely visualized normal-appearing appendix with no ancillary findings to suggest appendicitis
2	Partially visualized normal-appearing appendix with no ancillary findings to suggest appendicitis
3	Non-visualized appendix with no ancillary findings to suggest appendicitis
4	Equivocal
5a	Non-perforated acute appendicitis
5b	Perforated appendicitis

Source: Ref. [4].

Table 8.
Apply score.

examination, a normal appendix appears as a compressible and blind-ended tubular structure with a diameter smaller than 6 mm extending from the caecum. A lumen diameter greater than 6 mm with hyperechogenicity of the appendix mesentery fat and an appendiceal hyperemia in color Doppler or free fluid in the abdomen are all reliable sonographic signs of acute appendicitis. In CT scans these findings are similar but with a greater accuracy in the case of perforation where an abscess or a phlegmon are more clearly depicted [4, 33, 34].

Fallon and her colleagues developed the so-called Apply-score which is an ultrasound scoring system (**Table 8**) in children with suspected appendicitis. They studied and compared the results of the ultrasound findings in a pre- and post-implementation period of Apply-score. The results have shown a high sensitivity of 93%, a specificity of 92, 6% a positive predictive value of 85.1%, and a negative predictive value of 96.7%. These results are comparable to those in the pre-implementation period. Negative appendectomies rate did not change either. The most interesting observation of this study was that the rate of CT scan use decreased by 31%. The study concludes that the Apply-score is a reliable scoring system that can be used by all radiologists with very good results in diagnosing acute appendicitis in children [4].

7. Heidelberg score

A combination of clinical parameters and ultrasonography can lead to a more advanced scoring system that could diagnose simple and advanced appendicitis or even perforated appendicitis. Such an example is the Heidelberg Appendicitis Score (HAS) presented in 2017 and consists of four factors (continuous pain, tenderness in the right lower abdomen, rebound tenderness, ultrasound findings positive for appendicitis). This study included 157 children younger than 16 years old who presented with right lower quadrant pain. Its sensitivity in identifying appendicitis was 91% and its specificity was 93.8%. The most interesting finding was that this scoring system had a 100% negative predictive value which means that a negative HAScore excludes perforation and it is possible to identify perforation within children with appendicitis with a sensitivity of 77% and 100% specificity. The results of this study were better than other studies in children which used only ultrasound scans or the sum of clinical and laboratory parameters such as abdominal pain duration and CRP in order to distinguish simple from perforated appendicitis [35].

8. Complicated appendicitis in children

As it is mentioned above, for centuries it was thought that appendicitis was a progressive disease-causing peritonitis or intraabdominal abscess through a process of inflammation, necrosis, and perforation of appendix layers. Recently studies have confirmed the concept of two distinct pathological entities of appendicitis with different causes and prognosis: simple non-perforated appendicitis and complicated appendicitis.

In complicated appendicitis (pathologically defined as necrotic or gangrenous appendicitis with or without wall rupture), the appendix macroscopically is highly hyperemic, friable, with a wall in shades of violet, green, or even black. In some cases, there is a macroscopic rupture of the wall with intraluminal pus. Complicated appendicitis is always found with inflammation and necrosis of its layers, abscess formation, and thrombosis. The main characteristic finding is the necrosis of all layers of the wall. On the other hand, in simple inflammatory appendicitis, macroscopically, the appendix is congested, with an increased edematous diameter, while hyperemic obliteration of the vessels is observed, as well as pus or fibrinous exudates in its wall. Microscopic findings consist of polymorphonuclear infiltration of the layers, the presence of mucosal ulcers or thrombi, and the presence or absence of purulent or fibrinous exudate. If a foreign body is present in the lumen of the appendix, intense stimulation of giant cells and hyperproduction of mucus is observed [36, 37].

These pathological features can explain the different responses of some children with appendicitis in the studies where the conservative treatment (only antibiotics) is chosen. Simple appendicitis can be treated successfully with antibiotics in 92% of cases, thus complicated appendicitis proceeds rapidly to perforation in children in spite of conservative treatment. If from the very beginning the patients with complicated not perforated appendicitis are misdiagnosed as acute appendicitis patients and are chosen for antibiotic therapy they can have complications as the conservative therapy with antibiotics has failed.

That is why distinguishing the two entities of appendicitis is very important from the very beginning. Today in twenty-first century both for the doctor and the patient the best treatment must be chosen regarding not only the disease but also the patient. The surgeon should choose the best management with fewer complications for each patient. For the last 5 years the whole pediatric community has been searching for new scores or using the old ones to distinguish one entity of appendicitis from the other in simple cost-effective ways.

In 2020 Feng et al. presented a clinical prediction model for complicated appendicitis in children younger than 5 years of age. In a retrospective study of 382 children, Feng developed a prediction model that included age, white blood cell count, and duration of symptoms. In the validation sample, this model exhibited a high degree of discrimination (area under the curve [AUC]: 0.830, 95% confidence interval [CI]: 0.762–0.885). It was also compared with PAS and Alvarado scores and it was found that it could identify children at high risk for complicated appendicitis better than the above two scores. The study concluded that this model might be used to aid the differentiation of acute and complicated appendicitis for optimal treatment strategy [38].

In 2021 Pogorelic et al. evaluated the validity of appendicitis inflammatory response (AIR) score in differentiating complicated from simple (non-perforated) appendicitis in children. In a prospective observational study of 184 pediatric patients is concluded that the AIR score can differentiate perforated from non-perforated appendicitis in children with a high level of accuracy. In the AIR score, a cut-off value of 9 was demonstrated to serve as a reliable indicator of perforated appendicitis with a sensitivity and a specificity of 89.5 and 71.9%, respectively (AUC = 0.80; 95% CI: 0.719–0.871; p < 0.001) [39].

In 2022 Fujii and his team used the PAS score in a retrospective study including 161 patients aged <16 years to investigate its efficacy in predicting complicated appendicitis. This study showed that alone PAS is not a good predictor for complicated appendicitis. Thus, a PAS score >8 combined with the duration of symptoms >1 day and C-reactive protein level >4 mg/dl had a high specificity of 99%, a positive predictive value of 98%, and in the ROC curve an area under the curve of 0.91. The authors concluded that the combination of these three parameters is predictor of complicated appendicitis in children [40].

Another retrospective study published in 2023 by Byun and his team established a new algorithm for predicting complicated appendicitis in children based on CT scans and clinical features. This study included 315 children <18 years with acute appendicitis. The algorithm included CT findings such as transverse appendix diameter of >91.25 mm, intraluminal appendiceal air, intraluminal appendicolith, suspicious wall defect, ascites, periappendiceal infiltration, abscess or inflammatory mass, free air in the abdomen, WBC count, neutrophil count, CRP level and erythrocyte sedimentation rate (ESR). The AUC, sensitivity, and specificity of the diagnostic algorithm comprising features were 0.91 (95% CI, 0.86–0.95), 91.8% (84.5–96.4), and 90.0% (82.4–95.1) in the development cohort, and 0.7 (0.63–0.84), 85.9% (75.0–93.4), and 58.5% (44.1–71.9) in test cohort, respectively [41].

9. Complicated apendicitis pediatric score (CoApP)

As it has been clear clinical score systems such as PAS and Alvarado Score have the potential to correctly stratify children at low risk of acute appendicitis but they cannot predict which children should proceed directly to surgery. For this reason, in all intermediate or high-risk patients preoperative ultrasound and/or low-dose CT scan imaging is used. Ultrasound scan imaging demonstrates a high specificity but lower sensitivity for complicated appendicitis. In the literature, it has been reported that 56% of perforated appendicitis did not exhibit the typical imaging findings and these cases are misdiagnosed. In addition, conventional simulated CT scan imaging fails to detect 79.5% of gangrenous non-perforated appendicitis because these cases are misdiagnosed as uncomplicated appendicitis. Therefore, if conservative treatment is chosen for these complicated cases it will be a higher rate of treatment failure and severe complications.

In 2022 Tzortzopoulou et al. present a new score for complicated appendicitis (CoApP Score) in children. Our prospective observational study enrolled two cohorts of patients 5–15 years old. 407 consecutive patients were enrolled in the derivation cohort. The jumping-up test, preoperative laboratory, imaging, and histopathology data were collected. The score was validated in a separate cohort of 312 consecutive patients who were classified according to their risk of complicated appendicitis. A positive jumping-up test, vomiting, White Blood Cell count >13.5 x 10^{-3}/ml, lymphocytes <18% and C- reactive protein >50 mg/dl were the predictors for complicated appendicitis. The final prediction model (CoApPScore) exhibited an area under the curve (AUC) of 0.890 (95% CI: 0.859–0.922) [42, 43], (**Tables 9** and **10**).

With the CoApP Score patients with suspected acute appendicitis can be classified into three groups: high-risk group patients (score 6–7) who have 86.15% probability of complicated appendicitis and should be managed immediately. Intermediate group

	Optimal cut-off point	Sensitivity (%)	Specificity (%)	PPV (%)	NPV (%)	+ LR	- LR
Prediction model	0.62	76.8	89.2	88.7	77.6	7.11	0.26
ALVARADO score	7	57.3	79.7	64.3	67.2	2.83	0.54
PAS	7	64.6	70.3	70.7	64.2	3.52	0.61

Table 9.
Prediction model, ALVARADO score, and PAS performance at optimal cut-off point values (validation sample: n = 156).

Predictors	Score
Jumping-up test +ve	3
Vomitus	1
WBC count greater than 13.50 (x 10^{-3} μL)	1
LY (%) lower than 18	1
CRP greater than 50 mg/dL	1
Maximum score	7

WBC: White Blood Cells.
LY: Lymphocytes.
CRP: C-Reactive Protein.

Table 10.
The CoApPS score.

patients (score 4–5) have a 45% probability of complicated appendicitis and a 33% probability of simple appendicitis. For the best management of these patients, we suggest an abdominal ultrasound to differentiate complicated from simple appendicitis for the best management of the patients. The last group is low-risk group (score 0–3). Patients in this group have an 11.1% probability of complicated appendicitis and a 20.2% probability of simple appendicitis which could be managed conservatively with antibiotics and 24–48 hours of observation in the hospital or at home. Describing the potential utility of the CoApP Score, emergency ultrasound imaging would have been postponed in 14.5% of patients (p = 0.0016) and emergency negative explorations would have been cut by 87% [42].

In conclusion, stratifying RLQ pain patients with CoApP scores at the emergency department can guide even the most inexperienced doctors in making the right choice for emergency surgery or antibiotics-first management. CoApPS could be proved advantageous since it favors a timely intervention with potentially lower complications, length of stay, cost, and lost days from school. Prompt and correct diagnosis of complicated appendicitis will allow us to make the best decisions regarding safer patient care, balanced with fair management of hospital imaging resources [42].

10. Conclusion

In children, the appendix is not a nonfunctional organ left in the body. The appendix is not only a "storage pool" for the gut microbiota to balance the steady state of anti-inflammatory activities of the intestine but also its high content of lymphoid tissue (lymphocyte CD8+ T cells) plays an important role in the immune function of the body. That is the reason why nowadays conservative therapy for acute appendicitis must also be an option in the management of the disease.

As it is mentioned above acute appendicitis has two distinct pathological entities with different causes and prognosis: simple non-perforated appendicitis and complicated appendicitis. Only for simple appendicitis conservative management is ideal, thus complicated appendicitis could cause life-threatening conditions for children if we do not remove the appendix.

Distinguishing these two entities should be pediatric surgeon's priority nowadays. Diagnostic scores could help us first incorrect diagnosis of appendicitis and then distinguish between simple and complicated appendicitis in order to choose the right therapy for each patient. Furthermore, we could minimize complications and have a better and cost-effective nouveau in our patient's health management.

Author details

Adelais K. Tzortzopoulou
Consultant Pediatric Surgeon, 2nd Surgical Department, "P. & A. Kyriakou" Children's Hospital, Athens, Greece

*Address all correspondence to: t.k.adelais@gmail.com

IntechOpen

© 2025 The Author(s). Licensee IntechOpen. This chapter is distributed under the terms of the Creative Commons Attribution License (http://creativecommons.org/licenses/by/4.0), which permits unrestricted use, distribution, and reproduction in any medium, provided the original work is properly cited.

References

[1] Benabbas R, Hanna M, Sha J. Diagnostic accuracy of history, physical examination, laboratory tests and point-of care ultrasound for pediatric acute appendicitis in the emergency department: A systematic review and met-analysis. Academic Emergency Medicine. 2017;**5**:24. DOI: 10.1111/acem.13181

[2] Alvarado A. A practical score for the early diagnosis of acute appendicitis. Annals of Emergency Medicine. 1986;**15**:557-564. DOI: 10.1016/s0196-0644(86)80993-3

[3] Di Saverio S, Birindelli A, Kelly MD, et al. WSES Jerusalem guidelines for diagnosis and treatment of acute appendicitis. World Journal of Emergency Surgery : WJES. 2016;**11**:34. DOI: 10.1186/s13017-016-0090-5

[4] Fallon SC, Orth RC, Guillerman RP, Munden MM, Zhang W, et al. Development and validation for an ultrasound scoring system for children with suspected acute appendicitis. Pediatric Radiology. 2015;**45**(13):1945-1952. DOI: 10.1007/s00247-015-3443-4

[5] Samuel M. Pediatric appendicitis score. Journal of Pediatric Surgery. 2002;**37**:877-881. DOI: 10.1053/jpsu.2002.32893

[6] Bhangu A, Soreide K, Di Saverio S, Assarsson JH, Drake FT. Acute appendicitis: Modern understanding of pathogenesis, diagnosis, and management. Lancet. 2015;**386**:1278-1287. DOI: 10.1016/S0140-6736(15)00275-5

[7] Chung PHY, Dai K, Yang Z, et al. Validity of Alvarado score in predicting disease severity and postoperative complication in pediatric acute appendicitis. World Journal of Pediatric Surgery. 2018;**2**:e000003. DOI: 10.1136wjps-2018-000003

[8] Ohle R, Oreilly F, Obrien KK, Fahey T, Dimitrov BD. The Alvarado score for predicting acute appendicitis: A systematic review. BMC Medicine. 2011;**9**:139. DOI: 10.1186/1741-7015-9-139

[9] Peyvasteh M, Askarpour S, Javaherizadeh H, Besharati S. Modified Alvarado score in children with diagnosis of appendicitis. Arquivos Brasileiros de Cirurgia Digestiva. 2017;**30**(1):51-52. DOI: 10.1590/0102-6720201700010014

[10] Shogilev DJ, Duus N, Odom SR, Shapiro NI. Diagnosing appendicitis: Evidence- based review of the diagnostic approach in 2014. The Western Journal of Emergency Medicine. 2014;**15**(7):859-871. DOI: 10.5811/westjem.2014.9.21568

[11] Goncalves JP, Cerqueira A, Martins S. The Alvarado score validation in diagnosing acute appendicitis in children at Braga Hospital. Acta Médica Portuguesa. 2011;**24**(S2):583-588

[12] Heineman J. An evaluation of the Alvarado score as a diagnostic tool for appendicitis in children. Emergency Medicine Journal. 2012;**29**(12):1013-1014. DOI: 10.1136/emermed-2012-202054.2

[13] Schneider C, Kharbanda A, Bachur R. Evaluating appendicitis score systems using a prospective pediatric cohort. Annals of Emergency Medicine. 2006;**12**(16):778-784. DOI: 10.1016/j.annemergmed.2006.12.016

[14] Pogorelic Z, Rak S, Mrklic I, Juric I. Prospective validation of Alvarado and Pediatric Appendicitis score for the

diagnosis of acute appendicitis in children. Pediatric Emergency Medicine Journal. 2015;**31**:164-168. DOI: 10.1097/PEC.0000000000000375

[15] Sayed AO, Zeidan NS, Fahmy DM, Ibrahim HA. Diagnostic reliability of pediatric appendicitis score, ultrasound and low-dose computed tomography scan in children with suspected acute appendicitis. Therapeutics and Clinical Risk Management. 2017;**13**:847-854. DOI: 10.2147/TCRM.S134153

[16] Dingemann J, Ure B. Imaging and the use of scores for the diagnosis of appendicitis in children. European Journal of Pediatric Surgery. 2012;**22**(3):195-200. DOI: 10.1055/s-0032-1320017

[17] Hao TK, Chung NT, Huy HQ, et al. Combining ultrasound with a pediatric appendicitis score to dinstinguish complicated from uncomplicated appendicitis in a pediatric population. Acta Informatica Medica. 2020;**28**(2):114-118. DOI: 10.5455/aim.2020.28.114-118

[18] Kim DY, Shim DH, Cho KY. Use of the pediatric appendicitis score in a community hospital. Indian Pediatrics. 2016;**53**(3):217-220. DOI: 10.1007/s13312-016-0823-2

[19] Prada Arias M, Salgado Barreira A, Montero Sanchez M, Fernandez Eire P, Garcia Saavedra S, et al. Appendicitis versus non-specific acute abdominal pain: Pediatric appendicitis score evaluation. Anales de Pediatría (Barcelona, Spain). 2018;**88**(1):32-38. DOI: 10.1016/j.anpedi.2017.01.006

[20] Ebell MH, Shinholser J. What are the most clinically useful cut-offs for the Alvarado and Pediatric Appendicitis scores? A systematic review. Annals of Emergency Medicine. 2014;**64**(4):365-372.e2. DOI: 10.1016/jannemergmed.2014.02.025

[21] Song CW, Kang JW, Kim JY. Different clinical features and lower scores in clinical scoring systems for appendicitis in preschool children: Comparison with school age onset. Pediatric Gastroenterology, Hepatology and Nutrition. 2018;**21**(1):51-58. DOI: 10.5223/pghn.2018.21.1.51

[22] El-Shamy A. Prognostication of pediatric appendicitis with three scoring systems. Life Science Journal. 2017;**14**(6):17-24

[23] Bhatt M, Joseph L, Ducharme FM, Dougherty G, McGillivray D. Prospective validation of the pediatric appendicitis score in a Canadian Pediatric Emergency Department. Academic Emergency Medicine. 2009;**16**:591-596. DOI: 10.1111/j.1553-2712.2009.00445.x

[24] Andersson MH, Shinholser J, Andersson RE. Validation of the appendicitis inflammation response (AIR) score. World Journal of Surgery. 2021;**45**(7):2081-2091. DOI: 10.1007/s00268-021-06042-2

[25] Murphy CG, Glickman JN, Tomczak K, Wang YY, Beggs AH, et al. Acute appendicitis is characterized by a uniform and highly selective pattern of inflammatory gene expression. Mucosal Immunology. 2008;**1**(4):297-308. DOI: 10.1038/mi.2008.13

[26] Macco S, Vrouenraets BC, de Castro SM. Evaluation of scoring system in predicting acute appendicitis. Surgery. 2016;**160**(6):1599-1604. DOI: 10.1016/j.surg.2016.06.023

[27] Vaziri M, Nafissi N, Jahangiri F, Nasiri M. Comparison of the appendicitis inflamatory response and Alvarado scoring systems in the diagnosis of

acute appendicitis in children. Journal of Medicine and Life. 2021;**14**(1):75-80. DOI: 10.25122/jml-2020-0031

[28] Attia J. Moving beyond sensitivity and specificity: Using likehood ratios to help interpret diagnostic tests. Australian Prescriber. 2003;**6**:11-113. DOI: 10.18773/austprescr.2003.082

[29] Maguire J, Kulik D, Laupacis A, et al. Clinical prediction rules for children. A Systematic Review. 2011;**128**:666-677. DOI: 10.1542/peds.2011-0043

[30] Linnet K, Bossuyt PMM, KEM M, Reitsma JB. Quantifying the accuracy of a diagnostic test or marker. Clinical Chemistry. 2012;**58**(9):1292-1301. DOI: 10.1373/clnchem.2012.182543

[31] Kulik DM, Uleryk EM, Fan-Maguire JJ. Does this child has appendicitis? A systematic review of clinical prediction rules for children with acute abdominal pain. Journal of Clinical Epidemiology. 2013;**66**(1):95-104. DOI: 10.1016/j.jclinepi.2012.09.004

[32] Andersson RE. The natural history and tranditional management of appendicitis revisited: Spontanous resolution and predominance of prehospital perforations imply that a correct diagnosis is more important than an early diagnosis. World Journal of Surgery. 2007;**31**(1):86-92. DOI: 10.1007/s00268-006-0056-Y

[33] Smith MP, Katz DS, Lalani T, Carucci LR, Cash BD, et al. ACR appropriateness criteria right lower quadrant pain-suspected appendicitis. Ultrasound Quarterly. 2015;**31**(2):85-91

[34] Srinivasan A, Servaes S, Pena A, Darge K. Utility of CT after sonography fot suspected appendicitis in children: integration of a clinical scoring system with a staged imaging protocol. Emergency Radiology. 2015;**22**(1):31-42

[35] Boettcher M, Breil T, Gunther P. The Heidelberg appendicitis score simplifies identification of pediatric appendicitis. Indian Journal of Pediatrics. 2016;**83**(10):1093-1097. DOI: 10.1007/s12098-016-2106-2

[36] Carr NJ. The pathology of acute appendicitis. Annals of Diagnostic Pathology. 2000;**4**:46-58. DOI: 10.1016/s1092-9134(00)90011-x

[37] Zimmermann A. Appendicitis: Histopathology and classification. Progress in Surgery. 1998;**25**:18-26. DOI: 10.1159/000075515

[38] Feng W, Zhao XF, Li MM, Cui HL. A clinical prediction model for complicated appendicitis in children younger than five years of age. BMC Pediatrics. 2020;**20**:401. DOI: 10.1186/s12887-020-02286-4

[39] Pogorelic Z, Mihanovic J, Nincevic S, Luksic B, Baloevic SE, Polasek O. Validity of appendicitis inflammatory response score in distinguishing perforated from non-perforated appendicitis in children. Children (Basel). 2021;**8**(4):309. DOI: 10.3390/children8040309

[40] Fujii T, Tanaka A, Katami H, Shimono R. Applying the pediatric appendicitis score to predict complicated appendicitis in children. Pediatrics International. 2022;**64**(1):e14918. DOI: 10.1111/ped.14918

[41] Byun J, Park S, Hwang SM. Diagnostic algorithm based on machine learning to predict complicated appendicitis in children using ct, laboratory and clinical features. Diagnostics (Basel). 2023;**13**(5):923. DOI: 10.3390/diagnostics13050923

[42] Tzortzopoulou AK, Tsolia M, Spyridis N, Giamarelou P, Sfakiotaki R, Passalides A, et al. A new score for the diagnosis of complicated appendicitis in children—Complicated appendicitis pediatric score. Journal of Indian Association of Pediatric Surgeons. 2022;**27**(4):410-418. DOI: 10.4103/jiaps.jiaps_110_21. Epub 2022 Jul 26

[43] Tzortzopoulou AK, Giamarelou P, Tsolia M, Spyridis N, Vakaki M, Passalides A, et al. The jumping up (J-Up)test: Making the diagnosis of acute appendicitis easier in children. Global Pediatric Health. 2019;**6**:2333794X19884824. DOI: 10.1177/2333794X19884824

Chapter 6

Trends in Acute Appendicitis in Children

Lokadolalu K.R. Shanbhogue and Hesham Sayed Ahmad

Abstract

Acute appendicitis is a common surgical emergency in children, diagnosis can be challenging, especially in younger children. Physical examination, laboratory tests, and imaging are used to confirm the condition. Treatment usually involves an appendectomy, but delayed diagnosis can lead to complications such as perforation or abscess formation. Nonoperative management has increased in recent years, it is safe, but appropriate selection of patients is important. Most cases of appendectomy are now performed laparoscopically. In delayed cases, complications can be high.

Keywords: acute appendicitis, scoring system, perforated appendicitis, nonoperative management, laparoscopic appendectomy, intra-abdominal collection, chronic appendicitis

1. Introduction

Earlier in history, appendicitis was referred to as perityphlitis. In 1886, pathologist Reginald Fits described perityphlitis as due to inflammation of the appendix and introduced the term "appendicitis." He also predicted that the treatment for this condition would be surgical.

Abdominal pain in children is the most common reason for emergency department visits, with acute appendicitis accounting for about 30–40% of childhood admissions for abdominal pain. Appendicitis remains the most common acute surgical condition in this population [1].

2. Anatomy

The base of the appendix arises at the confluence of the three taeniae coli, which serve as useful landmarks for locating the appendix. Its width is typically normal up to 6 mm. In 95% of cases, the appendix is located in an intraperitoneal position, with 30% found in the pelvis and 65% in the retrocecal position; in 5% of cases, it is retroperitoneal. The blood supply to the appendix comes from the appendiceal branch of the ileocolic artery.

3. Etiology

Appendicitis results from obstruction of the lumen, with potential causes including lymphoid hyperplasia, fecaliths, parasites, foreign bodies, and, occasionally, a carcinoid tumor. There is a relationship between the incidence of appendicitis and the development of submucosal lymphoid follicles, which increase with age, peaking in adolescence. The incidence of fecaliths in pathologic specimens is as follows: 1.2% in negative appendicitis, 7% in acute appendicitis, and 12% in perforated appendicitis [2].

4. Clinical presentation

The classic presentation of appendicitis, which is not very common, is periumbilical pain that mitigates to the right iliac fossa over 12 hours, accompanied by anorexia, nausea, low-grade fever, and leukocytosis. Periumbilical pain originates viscerally due to distention of the appendix, which activates T-10 visceral nerve fibers. As inflammation becomes localized, somatic pain fibers in the parietal peritoneum are activated, causing pain in the right iliac fossa.

Anorexia is the second most common symptom, present in 90% of patients. Nausea and vomiting follow the onset of pain in around 60% of cases, though these are not reliable findings. Most children with appendicitis have a low-grade fever; however, a temperature above 39°C, is rare unless there is appendiceal rupture with peritoneal contamination. A high fever without peritoneal signs may suggest viral gastroenteritis or a urinary tract infection (UTI).

The anatomical variability of the appendix can significantly influence symptom presentation. For example, retrocecal appendicitis can cause inflammation of the ureter resulting in renal colic-type symptoms. Pelvic appendicitis may cause urinary frequency, diarrhea, and even referred testicular pain. Diarrhea is more commonly associated with perforated appendicitis, where small, frequent stools may occur. In contrast, large, foul-smelling stools are typical of gastroenteritis. Differentiating between the two is often based on pain localization; abdominal pain in gastroenteritis is diffuse and typically accompanied by repeated episodes of vomiting and diarrhea that start simultaneously or precede the onset of pain.

4.1 Diagnosis

A careful history, thorough physical examination, analysis of selected laboratory studies, and, in some cases, ultrasonography (US) or computed tomography (CT) scanning are essential for accurate diagnosis.

4.2 Physical examination

Serial examinations by the same examiner are important, as they allow for better assessment of changes over time. Patients often lie quietly with minimal movement; older patients may limp or flex their trunk to alleviate discomfort. Examining small children requires patience and experience, and can be challenging.

During examination, the patient's knees should be flexed to relax the abdominal muscles, making the abdomen softer and easier to palpate. The patient should be asked to point with one finger to the area of greatest tenderness, and the right lower quadrant (RLQ) should be examined last.

The examiner should begin with percussion, followed by shallow and gentle palpation to identify signs of peritoneal irritation. Rebound tenderness, assessed by pressing deeply in the RLQ and then rapidly releasing, is associated with an increased likelihood of appendicitis, though other peritoneal signs in children are often nonspecific.

Peritoneal signs include:

- Rovsing sign; Palpation of the lower left quadrant (LLQ) produces pain the RLQ
- Psoas sign: Pain elicited by right hip extension or by raising the straight leg against resistance
- Obturator sign: Pain with passive internal rotation of the right thigh

Rectal examination may reveal a palpable, tender mass; however, it is not routinely performed because it may not be acceptable to young patients and is nonspecific. Even in cases of suspected pelvic abscess or ovarian pathology, imaging is necessary for confirmation.

Bowel sounds are nonspecific and may vary depending on the condition. They are often absent in cases of perforation but hyperactive in gastroenteritis. In young children, a stethoscope can serve as a tool to gently palpate the abdomen to identify areas of tenderness.

5. Laboratory tests

In general, laboratory tests are neither highly sensitive nor specific for diagnosing appendicitis. Leukocyte counts are often mildly elevated (10,000-15,000/mm3), and the presence of a left shift can improve sensitivity. However, a normal leukocyte count does not exclude appendicitis. In children younger than 4 years, leukocytosis is more common and tends to decrease with age [3].

C-reactive protein (CRP) is used as a diagnostic aid, with sensitivity and specificity similar to those of leukocyte counts. When both WBC and CRP levels are normal, the likelihood of appendicitis is very low [2].

Electrolytes are not routinely measured, but preoperative hyponatremia is a useful tool for predicting the severity of appendicitis. Studies have shown that serum sodium levels are significantly lower in complicated appendicitis compared to uncomplicated cases. Preoperative serum sodium levels less than 135 mmol/L are associated with a high likelihood of gangrenous or perforated appendicitis, with good sensitivity and specificity [4, 5].

A urine dipstick test is quick way to evaluate urine; appendicitis near the ureter may cause mild hematuria and/or pyuria. In patients with periumbilical abdominal pain and repeated vomiting, serum amylase levels should be measured to exclude pancreatitis. Misdiagnosis and unnecessary surgical intervention can occur with quick examinations and rushed decisions.

5.1 Scoring system in acute appendicitis

Several scoring systems have been developed to aid in diagnosing appendicitis and reducing negative appendectomy rates. These include the Lintula scoring system, Alvarado score, Pediatric Appendicitis Score, modified Pediatric Appendicitis Score, and Tzanakis scoring system. These tools rely on a combination of symptoms, physical examination findings, and laboratory test results to stratify patients into low-, medium-, and high-risk categories to guide clinical management.

In a study comparing these scoring systems, it was found that the Lintula scoring system had the lowest rate of negative appendectomies, while the Tzanakis scoring system demonstrated the highest accuracy in diagnosing appendicitis [4, 6].

5.2 Differential diagnosis

The differential diagnosis of appendicitis includes a wide range of conditions such as constipation, gastroenteritis, mesenteric lymphadenitis, pancreatitis, Crohn's disease, Meckel's diverticulitis, ovarian torsion or cyst, intussusception, pyelonephritis, and renal stones.

It is important to note that certain systemic conditions, such as diabetic ketoacidosis and sickle cell anemia, can also present with acute abdominal pain and should be considered in the diagnostic process.

6. IMAGING in acute appendicitis

Ultrasound and CT scan are the main imaging modalities used for diagnosing acute appendicitis.

6.1 Ultrasonography

Ultrasound is a noninvasive imaging modality, but its accuracy depends heavily on the operator's expertise. Common ultrasonographic findings in appendicitis include a non-compressible, blind-ending tubular structure that is fluid-filled, with a diameter greater than 6 mm. Additional findings may include fecaliths, periappendiceal free fluid, and signs of inflammation such as increased echogenicity and fat stranding. Ultrasound has a sensitivity of approximately 85% and a specificity ranging from 89–98% [2, 7].

False negatives can occur, particularly in cases involving a retrocecal appendix or inflammation confined to the tip of the appendix. Ultrasound is particularly helpful in female patients to rule out gynecologic conditions like ovarian torsion and is also useful in diagnosing mesenteric lymphadenitis, which is common in children.

6.2 CT imaging

CT scanning is the diagnostic test of choice when the diagnosis is unclear, especially in obese patients, as it is more accurate than ultrasonography. Sensitivity and specificity are around 96 and 98%, respectively, [1, 8]. In general, CT is performed with IV contrast, but adding oral or rectal contrast can enhance sensitivity.

Key diagnostic criteria on CT include an appendix diameter greater than 6 mm, a non-opacified appendicular lumen, and marked wall enhancement. Minor findings include fat stranding, bowel wall thickening, and the presence of pus or fecaliths [9].

While CT is highly accurate, its use has not consistently reduced negative appendectomy rates. Concerns about radiation exposure, particularly in younger patients, and the associated risk of radiation-induced malignancy (estimated at 0.18% lifetime risk) suggest that routine CT use should be reevaluated [10]. Younger children have a higher risk of radiation from CT, but this risk decreases with age. The lifetime risk of fatal radiation-induced malignancy is 0.18% [2].

To minimize radiation exposure in children, it is recommended to use pediatric appendicitis score models and rely on ultrasound as the primary imaging modality. CT should be reserved for cases with inconclusive clinical, laboratory, and ultrasound findings [11, 12].

In our experience, we prioritize ultrasonography due to concerns about harmful radiation exposure and the need for conscious sedation or general anesthesia in younger children. CT scans are employed only when there is strong clinical suspicion of appendicitis but normal ultrasonographic findings.

6.3 Management

Appendicitis management can be categorized into nonoperative and operative approaches.

6.3.1 Nonoperative management of acute appendicitis

Although appendectomy is the treatment of choice for appendicitis, studies have shown that nonoperative management is safe and efficacious and does not increase the risk of complications. However, appropriate patient selection is critical and should include patients with a short duration of symptoms, radiologic confirmation of noncomplicated appendicitis, and no evidence of fecaliths [13]. Family should be included in the treatment decision.

A retrospective study reported an 85.6% success rate at 2 years for nonoperative management using antibiotics. The antibiotics used incluced IV Augmentin (amoxicillin-clavulanic acid, 80 mg/kg/day of amoxicillin) for the first 48 hours, followed by oral antibiotics for 5 days [14]. According to one study conducted during the COVID-19 pandemic, the risk of recurrence of appendicitis after nonoperative management was 24.3% over an average follow up period of 16.2 ± 4.7 months [15]. Another study in adults revealed recurrence rates of 27.3% at 1 year and 37.1% at 5 years in 257 patients treated with antibiotics for uncomplicated appendicitis [16].

In children, recurrence after nonoperative management is associated with a higher incidence of complicated appendicitis and increased postoperative complications [17]. The exact reasons for this remain unclear. In our experience, patients selected for nonoperative management based on their history, clinical examination, and ultrasound findings receive intravenous antibiotics for 48 hours. If their condition improves, they are discharged on oral antibiotics; otherwise, laparoscopic appendectomy is performed.

6.3.2 Operative management of acute appendicitis

Once the diagnosis of appendicitis is made, treatment begins with intravenous fluids and antibiotics. For nocomplicated appendicitis, a single preoperative dose of a broad-spectrum antibiotics (e.g., third-generation cephalosporin) is adequate. Postoperative antibiotics may be administered but are not routinely necessary. Triple antibiotics (ampicillin, gentamicin, and metronidazole or clindamycin) are still used in many centers [2]. A retrospective study found that a single dose of ceftriaxone (50 mg/kg/day) and metronidazole (30 mg/kg/day) is as effective as triple antibiotics, while being simpler and less expensive [2].

In complicated appendicitis, the length of time required for antibiotic treatment is still controversial. In our experience over the last 20 years, patients will continue IV antibiotics until leukocyte count normalizes and the patient is clinically well and afebrile. If the patient's condition improves clinically but the leukocyte count remains elevated, discharge with oral antibiotics is considered. Studies indicate that for children with perforated appendicitis, postdischarge antibiotics do not reduce surgical site infections or intra-abdominal abscess rates, suggesting it is safe to discharge patients once clinical criteria are met [18, 19].

Monotherapy with piperacillin/tazobactam has become the treatment of choice for intra-abdominal infections [2]. However, due to its high cost and frequent dosing requirements (3–4 doses per day), we reserve this option for patients unresponsive to ceftriaxone and metronidazole within 24–48 hours.

In the absence of generalized peritonitis, appendectomy is not an emergency once intravenous antibiotics are initiated. Most cases can safely be delayed until daylight hours [7].

6.4 Open vs. laparoscopic appendectomy

In the open approach, the abdomen is explored via transverse right lower quadrant incision (Rockey-Davis). The external fascia is opened, muscles are split, and the peritoneum is accessed. The appendix is delivered into the wound, the mesoappendix is tied and cut, and the appendiceal base is ligated and removed, with or without stump inversion (the outcomes are similar).

In the laparoscopic approach, three ports are used: a 10–12-mm port in the umbilical area (umbilical, supra or infra-umbilical incision), and two 5-mm ports in left mid-abdomen and suprapubic area. Diagnostic laparoscopy is performed initially to identify the appendix. The mesoappendix is ligated with a stapler or hook diathermy, and the appendiceal base is secured with an Endo loop. The appendix is removed, often in an endoscopic bag if it is too large. To minimize trocar site infections, the inflamed appendix should not contact the port sites.

In open or laparoscopic appendectomy, the use of drains is not useful except in cases with well-localized abscesses.

Several studies comparing laparoscopic and open appendectomy have been conducted.

Laparoscopic appendectomy offers several advantages, including better visualization of the abdominal cavity, lower rates of wound infection and adhesive bowel obstruction, reduced gastrointestinal complications, improved cosmetic outcomes, and greater comfort for obese patients [1–3, 7, 20]. In our practice, over 90% of appendectomies are performed laparoscopically, with a conversion rate of 2–3%. We find the laparoscopic approach feasible for all types of appendicitis, including perforated cases, with lower wound infection rates, reduced postoperative analgesia requirements, earlier resumption of feeds, and shorter hospital stays.

6.5 Perforated appendicitis

The risk of perforation increases in younger children, ranging from 15–20% in children aged 10–15 years to around 80% in children younger than 3 years [7, 21].

Patients with perforated appendicitis often present with prolonged symptoms, fever, elevated white blood cell counts, and diffuse abdominal tenderness. However, none of these factors, nor even CT scanning (unless a clear abscess is present), can accurately distinguish between perforated and nonperforated appendicitis. As a result, most perforated appendices are discovered during surgery.

If a well-defined abscess is diagnosed preoperatively through imaging, CT-guided drainage, intravenous antibiotics, and interval appendectomy are good options, offering a safer and less morbid approach. Regardless of whether the drainage is done percutaneously or during an open or laparoscopic procedure, culturing the fluid has not been shown to be helpful [2]. Interval appendectomy is typically performed 6–8 weeks later, with intravenous antibiotics continued until the patient becomes afebrile for 48 hours, tolerates oral feeding, and shows a normal white blood cell count. The patient can then be discharged on oral antibiotics for 1–2 weeks. However, both our own practice and recent studies suggest that early appendectomy, even in the presence of a localized abscess, may be a better option [2, 7].

6.5.1 Post-appendectomy complications

In general, uncomplicated appendicitis has low morbidity, while complicated appendicitis carries a significantly higher risk of postoperative complication. Patients with late presentation after 36–48 hours have a greater than 60% chance of complicated appendicitis, which increases over time [1]. The most common complications are surgical site infections, intra-abdominal collection, and adhesive intestinal obstruction. Less common complications include stump leakage and enterocutaneous fistula.

7. Intra-abdominal collection

The treatment approach is guided by location and size of abscess, availability of an interventional radiologist, and the patient's clinical condition. After diagnosing an intra-abdominal abscess, the patient should first be assessed for any signs of sepsis or even septic shock. In such cases, prompt evacuation (percutaneous or surgical) is needed. If the patient is stable, treatment depends on abscess size.

In general, all patients with abscess smaller than 3 cm are treated with noninvasive strategy. For a patient with a moderate size abscess (>6 cm), treatment starts with IV antibiotics for 48 hours. If symptoms improve and the patient remains stable, antibiotics can be continued. If there is no improvement, surgical or percutaneous drainage is required. For large abscesses (> 6 cm) or multiple abscesses, invasive treatment is preferred [22]. Studies have shown that antibiotic therapy alone can be an effective and safe firstline treatment, even in some cases of large abscesses [23].

In our experience, we administer IV antibiotics (piperacillin/tazobactam) to all patients with intra-abdominal abscesses, regardless of size, for 48 hours. if there is no response, the next step is percutaneous or surgical drainage.

In the absence of a reliable interventional radiologist, we have found that laparoscopic drainage of post-appendectomy abscesses offers better visualization, helps with irrigation and suctioning, and results in fewer operative complications.

7.1 Chronic appendicitis

Chronic appendicitis is chronic inflammation or fibrosis of the appendix. It is a rare condition, initially reported by Crymble and Forsythe in 1949 [24]. About 1.5%

of patients presenting with symptoms like acute appendicitis may have chronic appendicitis [25].

Clinically, chronic appendicitis presents as intermittent abdominal pain, typically mild to moderate, and often localized to the right iliac fossa. The pain can persist for months or even years. Systemic symptoms are usually absent, and laboratory tests often reveal a normal white blood cell count. Ultrasound may help identify other potential causes of abdominal pain.

Computed tomographic findings suggestive of chronic appendicitis include pericecal stranding, dilated appendix, apical thickening, and either a non-filling or partially filling appendix. Additionally, failure of contrast to drain from the appendix is another indicator of chronic appendicitis [1].

The management of chronic appendicitis involves laparoscopic exploration and appendicectomy if no other pathology is identified. A study reported that 70% of children with chronic abdominal pain experienced symptom relief following appendectomy [26].

In the differential diagnosis of a child with chronic abdominal pain, particularly in the RLQ, chronic appendicitis should be considered.

Author details

Lokadolalu K.R. Shanbhogue* and Hesham Sayed Ahmad
Department of Pediatric Surgery, Maternity and Childrens Hospital,
Buraidah, Algassim, Saudi Arabia

*Address all correspondence to: ragu150454@gmail.com

IntechOpen

© 2025 The Author(s). Licensee IntechOpen. This chapter is distributed under the terms of the Creative Commons Attribution License (http://creativecommons.org/licenses/by/4.0), which permits unrestricted use, distribution, and reproduction in any medium, provided the original work is properly cited.

References

[1] Grosfeld JL, JAJ O'N, Fonkalsrud EW, Coran AG. Pediatric Surgery. 6th ed. Philadelphia: Mosby; 2006

[2] Holcomb GW, Murphy JP, Ostlie DJ. Aschcraft' Pediatric Surgery. Chapter (43). 5th ed. Philadelphia: Elsevier Health Sciences; 2010. pp. 549-556

[3] Rentea RM, St Peter SD. Pediatric appendicitis. The Surgical Clinics of North America. 2017;**97**(1):93-112

[4] Elgendy A, Khirallah MG, Elsawaf M, Hassan HS, Ghazaly M. Acute appendicitis in children: Is preoperative hyponatremia a predictive factor of perforation/gangrene? A prospective study. Pediatric Surgery International. 2023;**39**(1):281

[5] Messias B, Cubas I, Oliveira C, Hashimoto F, Mocchetti E, Ichinose T, et al. Usefulness of serum sodium levels as a novel marker for predicting acute appendicitis severity: A retrospective cohort study. BMC Surgery. 2023;**23**(1):312

[6] Sağ S, Basar D, Yurdadoğan F, Pehlivan Y, Elemen L. Comparison of appendicitis scoring systems in childhood appendicitis. Turkish Archives of Pediatrics. 2022;**57**(5):532-537. DOI: 10.5152/TurkArchPediatr.2022.22076

[7] Mattei P, editor. Fundamental of Pediatric Surgery. New York: Springer; 2011

[8] Arensman RM, Bambini DA, Almond PS, Adolv V. Pediatric Surgery. 2nd ed. Berlin: CRC Press; 2009

[9] Yi DY, Lee KH, Park SB, Kim JT, Lee NM, Kim H, et al. Accuracy of low dose CT in the diagnosis of appendicitis in childhood and comparison with USG and standard dose CT. Jornal de Pediatria. 2017;**93**(6):625-631

[10] Martin AE, Vollman D, Adler B, Caniano DA. CT scans may not reduce the negative appendectomy rate in children. Journal of Pediatric Surgery. 2004;**39**(6):886-890. DOI: 10.1016/j.jpedsurg.2004.02.034

[11] Kim I, Kwon H, Choi YJ, Kwak YH, Lee JH, Suh D, et al. Computed tomography scan usage when US results are non-diagnostic for suspected acute appendicitis in children. Medicine (Baltimore). 2020, 2020;**99**(36):e21961

[12] Sayed AO, Zeidan NS, Fahmy DM, Ibrahim HA. Diagnostic reliability of pediatric appendicitis score, ultrasound and low-dose computed tomography scan in children with suspected acute appendicitis. Therapeutics and Clinical Risk Management. 2017;**13**:847-854. DOI: 10.2147/TCRM.S134153

[13] Jumah S, Wester T. Non-operative management of acute appendicitis in children. Pediatric Surgery International. 2023;**39**(1):11

[14] Picard C, Abbo O, Munzer C, Ricco L, Dubois D, Lemoine C, et al. Non-operative treatment of acute appendicitis in children: Clinical efficacy of amoxicillin-clavulanic acid in a retrospective single-centre study. BMJ Paediatrics Open. 2023;7:e001855

[15] Tan APP, Yap T-L, Cheong YL, Rai R, Choo C, Ong C, et al. Conservative antibiotic treatment of pediatric acute uncomplicated appendicitis during the COVID-19 pandemic: A prospective comparative cohort study. Pediatric Surgery International. 2022;**39**(1):60

[16] Salminen P, Tuominen R, Paajanen H, Rautio T, Nordström P, Aarnio M, et al. Five-year follow-up of antibiotic therapy for uncomplicated acute appendicitis in the APPAC randomized clinical trial. Journal of the American Medical Association. 2018;**20**(12):1259-1265

[17] Lipsett SC, Monuteaux MC, Shanahan KH, Bachur RG. Nonoperative management of uncomplicated appendicitis. American Academy of Pediatrics. 2022;**149**:5

[18] Gordon AJ, Choi J-H, Ginsburg H, Kuenzler K, Fisher J, Tomita S. Oral antibiotics and abscess formation after appendectomy for perforated appendicitis in children. The Journal of Surgical Research. 2020;**256**:56-60. DOI: 10.1016/j.jss.2020.05.082

[19] Jen J, Hwang R, Mattei P. Post-discharge antibiotics do not prevent intra-abdominal abscesses after appendectomy in children. Journal of Pediatric Surgery. 2023;**58**(2):258-262. DOI: 10.1016/j.jpedsurg.2022.10.024

[20] Aziz O, Athanasiou T, Tekkis PP, Purkayastha S, Haddow J, Malinovski V, et al. Laparoscopic versus open appendectomy in children. Annals of Surgery. 2006;**243**(1):17-27

[21] Pearl RH, Hale DA, Molloy M, Schutt DC, Jaques DP. Pediatric appendectomy. Journal of Pediatric Surgery. 1995;**30**(2):173-178

[22] Gorter RR, Meiring S, van der Lee JH, Heij HA. Intervention not always necessary in post-appendectomy abscesses in children; clinical experience in a tertiary surgical centre and an overview of the literature. PMC Journal. 2016;**175**(9):1185-1191. DOI: 10.1007/s00431-016-2756-0

[23] Moreno-Alfonso JC, Caballero AM, Martínez AP. Antibiotic treatment of post-appendectomy abscesses in children, regardless of size: A twelve years' experience. Updates in Surgery. 2023;**75**(8):2267-2272

[24] Kim D, Butterworth SA, Goldman RD. Chronic appendicitis in children. Canadian Family Physician. 2016;**62**(6):e304-e305

[25] Shah SS, Gaffney RR, Dykes TM, Goldstein JP. Chronic appendicitis: An often forgotten cause of recurrent abdominal pain. The American Journal of Medicine. 2013;**126**(1):e7-e8

[26] Stringel G, Berezin SH, Bostwick HE, Halata MS. Laparoscopy in the management of children with chronic recurrent abdominal pain. Journal of the Society of Laparoscopic & Robotic Surgeons. 1999;**3**(3):215-219

Chapter 7

Decoding Pediatric Appendicitis: Unraveling Complexity with Artificial Intelligence and Evolving Management Insights

Anas Shikha and Asem Kasem

Abstract

Pediatric appendicitis poses unique diagnostic and management challenges, necessitating a precise approach that considers the complexities of developing anatomy and subtle clinical presentations. This chapter addresses these challenges by integrating clinical expertise with advanced technology, showcasing the potential of artificial intelligence models such as the artificial intelligence pediatric appendicitis decision-tree (AiPAD) to streamline diagnostic accuracy. In addition to improving decision-making, this chapter provides a comprehensive overview of the latest management strategies, offering valuable insights into optimizing outcomes and reducing complications. By bridging innovative AI techniques with evolving management principles, this chapter serves as a crucial resource for clinicians aiming to enhance their understanding and approach to pediatric appendicitis.

Keywords: pediatric appendicitis, decision tree (DT), AI-augmented clinical decision, artificial intelligence pediatric appendicitis decision-tree (AiPAD), nonoperative vs. operative management of appendicitis in children, enhanced recovery after surgery (ERAS), rationalizing the role of imaging studies

1. Introduction

Appendicitis is a common yet challenging inflammatory condition, particularly within the pediatric population. Given the rapid progression of the disease in children, timely diagnosis is critical to prevent serious complications. While advancements in imaging technology have improved diagnostic capabilities, clinical examination remains the cornerstone in identifying appendicitis in children, where the presentation differs markedly from adults, making traditional scoring systems often inadequate.

This chapter delves into the unique complexities of pediatric appendicitis, emphasizing the need for diagnostic approaches tailored specifically to younger patients.

IntechOpen

It also explores the transformative role of artificial intelligence (AI) in enhancing diagnostic accuracy, preserving essential clinical skills, and revolutionizing the training of future healthcare professionals. The ongoing debate between conservative management with antibiotics versus surgical intervention is also addressed, underscoring the need for a clear and validated framework to guide clinical decisions. By navigating these critical aspects, this chapter aims to equip healthcare professionals with the knowledge and tools to provide timely and effective care for pediatric appendicitis.

2. Unraveling the unique complexities of appendicitis in the pediatric patient

Appendicitis in children (under 12 years) exhibits distinct characteristics due to their developing anatomy, psychology, and immune system. These differences affect the disease's evolution, progression, and clinical presentation.

In contrast to the adult population, where fecal impaction is a common underlying cause of obstruction of the appendicular lumen, mucosal inflammation of the appendix is a more frequent etiology in children. This difference is related to the unique immunological activity in the pediatric population, where viral or bacterial infections can trigger intraluminal inflammation and infection [1, 2].

Anatomically, while the pediatric abdomen is smaller and less spacious, the position of the appendix in children can vary more widely than in adults, contributing to a less predictable clinical presentation [3]. The classic symptoms of right iliac fossa pain and migration of pain are less reliable in children, who often present with atypical symptoms such as vague or diffuse abdominal pain, dysuria, or diarrhea. These symptoms arise because the pelvis is shallower and the appendix in children may be located closer to the lower midline, neighboring the bladder or rectum, causing irritation of these adjacent organs. Furthermore, in younger children, the pain is often poorly localized, making the diagnosis of appendicitis more challenging.

The immune response in children is more complex and unpredictable due to the immaturity of their developing defense mechanisms. Generally, the immune system's response in children is more aggressive, leading to a rapid progression of appendicitis. However, children's ability to heal and recover is typically faster and more effective than adults [4]. For example, intra-abdominal defense mechanisms in children are weaker, the omentum is less developed, and the appendiceal wall is thinner, which increases the risk of perforation and rapid disease spread.

Children often struggle to perceive and communicate their pain, making it difficult to interpret symptoms directly from them. Instead, diagnosis relies heavily on observation by caregivers. This, combined with the unique features mentioned above, makes appendicitis in children a distinct entity from the adult form of the disease. However, as children approach adolescence, they are more likely to exhibit adult-like manifestations of appendicitis [5].

Adding to the complexities of diagnosing appendicitis in children is the presence of strong mimickers, such as mesenteric adenitis. Mesenteric adenitis, an inflammation of the mesenteric lymph nodes near the appendix, is common in children and often mimics the symptoms of appendicitis. The abdominal pain, nausea, and fever associated with mesenteric adenitis closely resemble the classic signs of appendicitis, making it challenging for clinicians to differentiate between the two.

Given the challenges of diagnosing appendicitis in children, the next sections will explore the clinical nuances of diagnosis, considering the unique aspects of abdominal pain in children. The authors will introduce a novel approach that combines clinical expertise with AI, allowing the insights of seasoned practitioners to be transferred to less experienced clinicians. This innovative method aims to enhance clinical decision-making, offering practitioners a precise, simplified, and experience-driven tool.

3. Mastering the diagnosis of pediatric appendicitis: A reorganized and focused approach

Early diagnosis of appendicitis in children is crucial for initiating timely treatment and preventing complications. Pediatric appendicitis can progress rapidly, and the diagnostic process is often complicated by the presence of alternative diagnoses. This section presents the author's philosophy and distilled experience, offering a structured and focused approach to diagnosing appendicitis in children. Emphasis is placed on real clinical scenarios where practitioners must not only identify appendicitis but also carefully consider and rule out other potential diagnoses.

3.1 Age-related diagnosis: Navigating the spectrum of causes

When evaluating a child with abdominal pain, structuring the differential diagnosis according to the child's age is the first critical step. This approach allows clinicians to prioritize the most likely causes and narrow down the possibilities efficiently. For example, in children under three years, intussusception is a more probable cause of abdominal pain than appendicitis. Between ages three and six, while appendicitis becomes more common, mesenteric adenitis remains a more frequent diagnosis. From ages seven to twelve, appendicitis becomes increasingly likely, especially when supported by other clinical findings. Recognizing this age-related spectrum is crucial for guiding the clinical assessment and improving diagnostic accuracy. **Table 1** summarizes the probable causes of abdominal pain in children based on their age.

Age group	1 to 3 years	4 to 6 years	7 to 12 years
The most common cause	Intussusception	Mesenteric adenitis	Appendicitis
Less frequent cause	Mesenteric adenitis	Appendicitis	Mesenteric adenitis
Rarer causes	Appendicitis	Intussusception Urinary stones Nephrotic syndrome	Urinary stones Ovarian torsion Testicular torsion
Other common, but easier-to-rule-out causes	Acute gastroenteritis Constipation Strangulated inguinal hernia Urinary tract infection		

Table 1.
Age-specific causes of abdominal pain in children.

3.2 The art of history-taking: Unlocking key diagnostic clues

History-taking is the cornerstone of diagnosis, offering invaluable clues while also establishing trust with both the child and their parents. It is crucial to dedicate sufficient time and attention to the parents, not only to gather information but also to ease their anxiety. The examiner should engage with the child by making eye contact, engaging in conversation (if verbal), smiling, and being cheerful before starting the physical examination, which helps to reduce anxiety for both the child and their parents.

3.2.1 The nature and duration of pain

Understanding the nature of the pain (colicky or constant) is essential in diagnosing the underlying condition. Colicky pain is characterized by intermittent and fluctuating intensity, often suggesting conditions where there is an obstruction or spasm, such as in intussusception, renal stones, or biliary colic. In contrast, constant pain is continuous and persistent, without significant fluctuations, often indicating inflammation or infection, as seen in appendicitis.

A child who prefers to stay still, avoiding movement, is likely experiencing peritonitis, where any movement exacerbates the pain. This is often caused by appendicitis, where the inflammation spreads to the peritoneum, causing severe, steady pain.

The duration of pain offers critical diagnostic insights. Appendicitis typically evolves over 12–24 hours, with the pain gradually worsening as the condition progresses. However, if the pain is sudden, severe, and appears earlier, it may indicate other conditions such as ovarian torsion, urinary stones, or intussusception. Pain lasting more than a week or recurring over several months is unlikely to be related to appendicitis, and functional pain should be considered in the differential diagnosis.

3.2.2 Vomiting, anorexia, and fever

The sequence of symptoms provides crucial diagnostic clues. In appendicitis, vomiting usually follows the onset of pain by several hours, which is a key indicator of the condition. In contrast, if vomiting precedes the pain, this pattern is more suggestive of acute gastroenteritis (AGE), particularly when accompanied by the onset of diarrhea.

The abrupt onset of vomiting coupled with severe colicky pain might indicate other conditions such as renal stones and ovarian torsion, where the pain is often intense and intermittent.

It is important to note that in young children with intussusception, vomiting may be less prominent or even absent. Therefore, the absence of vomiting should not exclude intussusception from the differential diagnosis, especially if other clinical findings point towards it.

Fever and anorexia in children with appendicitis are less consistent and reliable than in adults. Typically, fever may present as low-grade (<38.5°C) during the early stages. However, as the condition progresses or if perforation occurs, the fever may rise to a high-grade level, and anorexia may become more pronounced.

3.2.3 Bowel opening

Bowel habits offer significant diagnostic insights. For instance, a child with a prolonged history of constipation might be experiencing stool impaction causing abdominal pain. In contrast, a child with normal bowel habits who develops obstruction following the onset of abdominal pain may be facing an obstruction, possibly due to an inflamed appendix.

'Diarrhea', while often misleading, requires careful interpretation. Large, frequent stools typically indicate acute gastroenteritis (AGE), whereas small, frequent stools, with or without mucus, may suggest rectal irritation from an inflamed appendix located in the pelvis or even direct influence of appendicitis on the adjacent bowel.

3.3 Minimally disruptive examination: Precision with care

When examining a child's abdomen, it is important to recognize that typical signs used in adult patients, such as Rovsing's sign or rebound tenderness, are often less useful and can be distressing for children. These signs, intended to identify peritonitis or guarding, may not be necessary in pediatric patients because these findings can often be detected more easily due to the thinner abdominal wall in children.

The examination process essentially begins during history-taking through careful observation of the child's behavior. For example, a child who walks stooped holding his/her abdomen is likely exhibiting guarding, a sign of peritonitis. An irritable young child who refuses to be touched may be scared of being touched to avoid triggering the pain.

The child is positioned in a straight supine position and asked to point to the area of max tenderness (if verbal). It is crucial at this stage to observe whether the abdomen is 'breathing' or stiffened with only breathing chest as this is a sign of guarding where the abdominal muscles are stiffened to avoid eliciting the pain.

For the physical examination, a simple, swift, and minimally disruptive approach is recommended. After establishing trust during history-taking and informing the child and parents about the upcoming steps, gently palpate the abdomen starting away from the area of maximum tenderness. Use distraction techniques to help the child remain calm and to accurately identify guarding, which is the stiffening of the abdominal muscles. For uncooperative younger children, examining them while they are held by a caregiver may be appropriate. Guarding is best assessed over the lateral abdominal muscles, as the rectus muscles are naturally stiffer in children.

In cases where the appendix is deep in the pelvis, clinical signs may be subtle (vague lower abdominal pain) and may not become apparent until the disease has advanced. Thus, vigilance in history-taking is crucial. A rectal examination is generally unnecessary and can be extremely painful, especially in cases of deep pelvic appendicitis. Instead, a thorough history combined with a focused abdominal examination and suggestive laboratory findings should be sufficient to make an accurate diagnosis.

It is equally important to examine the pelvis thoroughly to identify any abnormalities that could suggest an alternative diagnosis. For instance, the pelvic inspection might reveal a strangulated inguinal hernia, epididymo-orchitis, torsion testis or posthitis, each of which can cause referred pain to the abdomen.

3.4 Laboratory insights: Supporting the clinical picture

Laboratory tests can complement the clinical findings. An elevated white blood cell (WBC) count with neutrophilia is the most reliable marker for appendicitis. C-reactive protein levels, while helpful, are less specific. Urinalysis is necessary when urinary symptoms are present; findings such as some WBCs and red blood cells (RBCs) in the absence of significant bacteriuria or nitrites can support a diagnosis of appendicitis.

3.5 Mimickers of appendicitis: Considering alternative diagnoses

When evaluating a child for appendicitis, it is essential to consider alternative diagnoses that may mimic its symptoms. For instance, a history of a recent upper respiratory tract infection or AGE could suggest mesenteric adenitis or, in rare cases, referred pain from lower lobe pneumonia. In children younger than 3 years, it is particularly important to rule out intussusception, as such infections can cause inflammation of Peyer's patches, which is a common precursor to this condition.

Urinary tract infections (UTIs) may also present with abdominal pain, but this is usually preceded by dysuria. In contrast, appendicitis might occasionally lead to dysuria, but this typically occurs a day or more after the onset of abdominal pain, which is more widespread across the lower abdomen. A urine analysis can offer additional clues to differentiate between these conditions.

Furthermore, underlying conditions such as IgA vasculitis (Henoch-Schönlein Purpura, or HSP) and nephrotic syndrome can present with abdominal pain that may be confused with appendicitis, particularly at their initial presentation. HSP is often associated with colicky abdominal pain, palpable purpura (commonly on the buttocks and legs), and may also be associated with intussusception. In contrast, nephrotic syndrome typically presents with diffuse abdominal pain, periorbital oedema, and significant proteinuria on urine analysis. Both HSP and nephrotic syndrome usually show no neutrophilia and likely have normal white blood cell counts.

3.6 Streamlining diagnosis: Fostering clinical judgment in the modern era

The refined and practical approach described above, which focuses on the most critical clinical findings, helps avoid the confusion that can arise from an exhaustive list of conflicting signs (**Table 2**). This approach is particularly beneficial for less experienced practitioners who may be overwhelmed by the pressures of managing a suffering child and anxious parents, compounded by the challenges of applying adult-based knowledge that is less relevant in pediatric cases. By concentrating on the essence of the diagnosis and avoiding the pitfalls of fitting numerous signs into an appendicitis scoring system, practitioners can build a solid foundation for recognizing positive and negative patterns that lead to sound clinical judgment. A well-trained clinician with a developed 'clinical sense' can often reach an accurate diagnosis swiftly without the need for imaging studies or extensive workup.

However, the current medical practice increasingly relies on scoring systems and imaging studies, such as ultrasonography (USG) and computed tomography (CT), often making these modalities nearly indispensable. This growing dependence on imaging has, in turn, led to a reduction in emphasis on clinical findings and may impede the development of essential clinical skills. This shift is partially attributable to a lack of experience and confidence in clinical diagnostic capabilities.

The forthcoming section will delve into how AI, particularly prediction models built using machine learning methods, could transform this landscape [6]. To ensure both practical utility and professional accountability, we emphasize the use of transparent models that offer explainable predictions, focusing specifically on machine learning decision tree (MLDT) models [7]. Imagine a tool that merges traditional

Parameter	Suggestive finding	Unlikely finding
Age	> 7 years	< 3 years
Nature of pain	Constant with slower progression	Sharp pain with sudden onset.
Duration of pain at presentation	12 to 24 hours	Less than 12 hours or more than 4 days
Vomiting	Starts a few hours after the pain	Starts acutely before or concomitant with abdominal pain
Bowel opening	Normal or obstipation	'Large' diarrhea or constipation
Associated illnesses	Nil	URTI, AGE, UTI, HSP, NPS
Location of max tenderness	Localized at the lower abdomen	Multiple locations including the upper and lower abdomen
Presence of guarding	Strong indicator if present	Absent
WBC	Elevated	Normal
Neutrophilia	Dominant	Normal or lymphocytosis
Urine analysis	Few WBC and RBC	Packed with WBC, bacteria, and positive nitrite. The presence of heavy proteinuria.

URTI: Upper Respiratory Tract Infection, AGE: Acute Gastroenteritis, UTI: Urinary Tract Infection, HSP: Henoch-Schönlein Purpura, NPS: Nephrotic Syndrome.

Table 2.
Indicators of appendicitis in children.

clinical expertise with advanced technology, turning novice practitioners into adept diagnosticians with remarkable speed. By providing a robust diagnostic pattern to identify or rule out appendicitis with minimal findings, MLDT promises to sharpen the diagnostic skills of junior doctors and reduce their reliance on imaging.

4. AI-enhanced clinical decision

4.1 From clinical intuition to data-driven precision: Harnessing neuronal plasticity and MLDTs in pediatric appendicitis diagnosis

The ability of a doctor to diagnose conditions with instinctual accuracy often stems from neuronal plasticity (NP), a process that enables the brain to adapt and reorganize itself through repeated exposure to specific tasks. This neural adaptation underpins the development of clinical expertise [8]. For example, when a trainee learns to diagnose abdominal pain in children, their brain is repeatedly stimulated by the variety of cases they encounter. This stimulation strengthens and reorganizes neural connections, enabling the trainee to differentiate between conditions such as appendicitis and non-appendicitis. Over time, these reinforced pathways consolidate into stable memories, forming the foundation of a 'clinical sense', an almost intuitive ability to make accurate diagnoses based on experience [9].

While this clinical 'sense' is powerful, it operates subconsciously and is difficult to articulate or standardize. Human intuition, though invaluable, remains subjective and challenging to teach. Here, MLDTs present a transformative opportunity, replicating and even enhancing this clinical intuition through data-driven and explainable decision-making models.

MLDTs mimic the learning process by analyzing vast datasets and identifying critical patterns essential for accurate diagnoses. Unlike the often inexplicable 'clinical sense' of human experts, MLDTs provide a transparent and explainable approach to decision-making. A prime example of this is the artificial intelligence pediatric appendicitis decision-tree (AiPAD) [7], which exemplifies the capabilities of MLDTs in diagnosing appendicitis in children, having been trained on meticulously curated datasets from an expert clinician.

AiPAD replicates the decision-making process for diagnosing appendicitis in children by analyzing expert-refined datasets from numerous cases. It identifies the most relevant clinical parameters (**Table 3**) and their diagnostic patterns, presenting them in a clear, rational decision tree (**Figure 1**). AiPAD not only achieves high accuracy (sensitivity of 96.7% and specificity of 97.4%) but also offers transparent explanations for each step in the diagnostic process, addressing the limitations of human intuition by providing a more standardized and reliable method of decision-making [7].

The integration of MLDTs like AiPAD into clinical practice represents a significant advancement. By combining the strengths of human expertise, the precision of machine learning algorithms, and the transparency of decision trees, MLDTs can deliver more accurate, unbiased, and explainable diagnostic decisions, ultimately leading to better patient care.

4.2 The difference between traditional scoring systems and machine learning decision trees in diagnosing appendicitis

Traditional scoring systems like Alvarado, RIPASA, PAS, and other modified versions have long been used to aid in diagnosing appendicitis. These systems rely on

AiPAD parameters
1. **Guarding**: Defined as the stiffening of the abdominal muscles, best assessed over the lateral abdominal wall (see Section 3.3). Proper distraction techniques should be employed during the examination. Guarding is considered positive if present during palpation, regardless of whether it is voluntary or involuntary, localized or generalized, to reduce subjectivity as much as possible.
2. **The Nature of Pain**: The nature of pain should be assessed through a thorough discussion with the patient and/or their parents. It is either **colicky** or **constant**. **Colicky**: Pain that comes and goes or varies significantly in intensity. In non-verbal children, this may present as the child appearing relatively well between episodes of crying or discomfort. **Constant**: Pain that is present continuously with a consistent intensity. In non-verbal children, it manifests as persistent discomfort affecting their usual activities, making the child appear consistently unwell.
3. **Tenderness is considered localized to the lower abdomen (positive)** if either the patient indicates the area of maximum tenderness or the examiner identifies it during palpation. If tenderness is present at multiple sites, including both the upper and lower abdomen, it is not considered localized to the lower abdomen (**negative**).
4. The Percentage of Neutrophils (%)
5. White Blood Cell Count (WBC 10^3 u/L)

Table 3.
Definition of critical parameters of AiPAD.

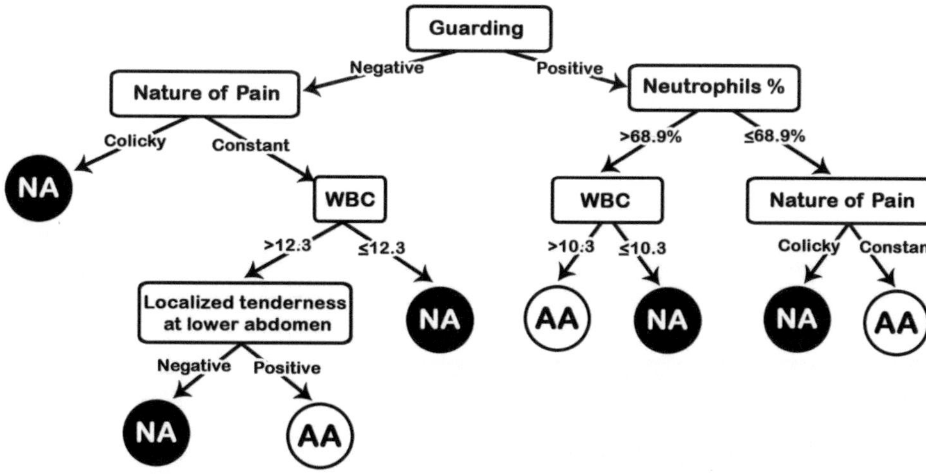

Figure 1.
Artificial intelligence pediatric appendicitis decision-tree (AiPAD). AA: acute appendicitis, NA: non-appendicitis, WBC: white blood cell count (10^3 u/L).

a set of predefined criteria, assigning scores to various clinical parameters to support or refute the diagnosis. However, they often incorporate irrelevant parameters, introducing 'noise' that can obscure decision-making and lead to inconsistencies. These systems are primarily effective in filtering extreme scores, while cases with intermediate scores typically require imaging studies for confirmation [10, 11].

In contrast, MLDTs offer a more refined approach by focusing only on the most critical parameters. For example, the AiPAD model, an MLDT specifically designed for diagnosing appendicitis, identified just five essential clinical parameters out of the fifteen available in the datasets. By concentrating on these five key factors, AiPAD significantly improves diagnostic accuracy [7]. However, while the remaining parameters were identified as non-critical in diagnosing appendicitis, they may still offer valuable clues for alternative diagnoses.

AiPAD and similar MLDTs address the variability in clinical practice by standardizing the diagnostic process. Different experts may prioritize different factors, leading to variations in diagnosis. MLDTs analyze data from various practitioners, identifying the most consistently important parameters to define a best-practice approach that reflects collective experience. This enhances diagnostic accuracy and promotes standardization across different clinical settings.

Traditional scoring systems often claim to provide highly accurate diagnoses, but these results can be inconsistent when tested on future or new patient populations [11, 12]. This inconsistency is often due to overfitting, where the system is too finely tuned to the specific data it was developed on, making it less effective with other datasets. The accuracy reported during development, known as 'training accuracy', might give an overly optimistic picture that does not hold up when tested on a new group of patients. AiPAD and other MLDTs tackle this issue using methods like cross-validation (XV), which helps ensure the model's predictions are consistent and reliable across unseen future datasets [13]. By rigorously developing and testing MLDT models with XV, we can reduce overfitting and achieve more trustworthy accuracy estimates, leading to dependable predictions for future patients. For example, AiPAD's XV estimated a negative predictive value (NPV) of 95.1 ± 2.9%. Although the training accuracy showed an NPV of 100%, when AiPAD was prospectively validated, the NPV was 97.4% matching the XV expectations [7]. Ultimately, accurately estimating the reliability of a model or scoring system is not just a technical detail, but it is fundamental to its practical use, acceptance, and overall effectiveness, ensuring that it can truly deliver dependable results in real-world scenarios.

4.3 Enhancing clinical decision-making in novice trainees with AiPAD

AiPAD exemplifies the potential of MLDTs in enhancing clinical decision-making, particularly for novice trainees. AiPAD encapsulates expert clinical judgment into an accessible and explainable model, significantly improving the diagnostic accuracy of trainees.

In a study conducted between March 2019 and October 2022, eight junior trainees in General Surgery and Pediatrics were tasked with diagnosing appendicitis in children using AiPAD. The results demonstrated a significant improvement in diagnostic accuracy when AiPAD was integrated into their decision-making process. On their own, trainees achieved an average accuracy rate of 70%, but with AiPAD, their accuracy increased to 97% [9].

The significant improvement in diagnostic accuracy highlights AiPAD's role in transforming novice decision-making, effectively bridging the gap to expert-level judgment. While traditional 'clinical sense' evolves over years of exposure, AiPAD accelerates this process, enabling trainees to tap into the distilled expertise of seasoned practitioners, significantly shortening the learning curve. This ensures a more reliable 'clinical sense', particularly in environments where trainees may not encounter a diverse range of cases or receive prolonged training.

Furthermore, AiPAD addresses the challenges of a culture heavily reliant on imaging studies, which can lead to reduced emphasis on clinical findings. By providing a decision-making framework that mirrors the judgment of an experienced surgeon, AiPAD supports trainees in making more accurate diagnoses, ultimately improving patient outcomes.

4.4 Implementing AiPAD for optimal diagnosis of pediatric appendicitis

To effectively utilize AiPAD's capabilities in children with suspected appendicitis, the author proposes that clinicians first apply the methodology for assessing abdominal pain as detailed in Section 3. Once this systematic approach has been followed, AiPAD (refer to **Table 3** and **Figure 1**) can then be applied to guide the next steps.

If AiPAD indicates a non-appendicitis diagnosis, the clinician should, by this stage, have gathered sufficient clues (as per the guidelines in Section 3) to direct further management and tailor investigations towards the most probable alternative diagnosis. Conversely, if AiPAD suggests appendicitis, management should be initiated promptly without additional imaging studies to avoid delays and associated complications.

Looking ahead, the authors envision that with more data and broader implementation of MLDT models, a comprehensive model could be developed that encapsulates the major causes of abdominal pain in children, extending beyond appendicitis alone. The upcoming section will further explore the author's perspective on the role of radiology in this context.

5. Rationalizing the application of imaging studies in diagnosing appendicitis

Over the past two decades, imaging studies, particularly USG and CT, have become increasingly prevalent in diagnosing appendicitis, especially in advanced pediatric centres. While USG is favored in pediatric settings due to its non-invasive nature and absence of ionizing radiation, it demands a high level of operator expertise to yield reliable results. In contrast, adult centres often rely on CT scans, which, though highly sensitive, expose patients to significant levels of radiation. This reliance on imaging raises concerns about potential overuse, given the associated risks, costs, availability, treatment delays, and the variability in diagnostic accuracy reported even with CT scans [14–19].

The accuracy of ultrasound (USG) in diagnosing appendicitis can vary significantly depending on the operator's experience, leading to potential false negatives or inconclusive results that may delay diagnosis or necessitate additional CT scans [18, 19]. While CT scans generally offer higher sensitivity, they are not without limitations, including the potential for misinterpretation [17] and the risks associated with radiation exposure, particularly in children [20–22].

Studies have shown that the false positive rate (FPR) for CT scans in children suspected of having appendicitis is about 12%, while the false negative rate (FNR) is approximately 16%, both of which raise concerns about CT being considered the 'gold standard' [14, 15]. Moreover, research has indicated that CT scans have not significantly reduced FPR or FNR in pediatric cases [14–16], and there are high rates of equivocal CT results, often necessitating a second review by a pediatric radiologist to improve accuracy [17]. The case for USG is even weaker, with higher FPR and FNR, even in the hands of experts [18, 19]. In contrast, the AiPAD model, which is purely based on clinical findings, has demonstrated an FPR of 2.6% and an FNR of 3.3%. Even the higher error estimates from cross-validation (FPR 8.2% and FNR 5.2%) remain superior to the reported rates for USG and CT [7]. Several other AI-based models have also been introduced recently, showing superior accuracy compared to USG and CT [6]. Based on this argument, the authors believe that achieving high diagnostic accuracy in appendicitis often hinges on a thorough clinical assessment supported by laboratory tests (Sections 3 and 4), rather than routine imaging. This approach not only minimizes the inherent challenges and risks of imaging but also cultivates essential clinical skills in trainees, an area increasingly neglected due to the rising dependence on radiological studies.

In this context, the authors believe that imaging should be reserved for cases where the clinical presentation is atypical or when alternative diagnoses need to be considered based on the clinical presentation. For instance, in children under three years old with colicky abdominal pain, an ultrasound is warranted to rule out intussusception, a leading cause of abdominal pain in this age group. In peri-pubertal girls or those with sudden onset of lower abdominal pain, ultrasound is crucial to exclude ovarian torsion, a surgical emergency often mistakenly attributed to appendicitis. Additionally, imaging is necessary when the clinical scenario is suggestive of urinary stones. Furthermore, in patients with septic shock, morbid obesity, neutropenia, or those who were on antibiotics, where traditional clinical signs of appendicitis may be unreliable, imaging becomes indispensable. These scenarios highlight the need for a rational, judicious approach to imaging, using it not to confirm or deny appendicitis, but mainly to consider or exclude other diagnoses.

Ultimately, the judicious application of imaging studies in appendicitis not only preserves the integrity of clinical training but also ensures that patients receive the most appropriate and least invasive care. By prioritizing clinical judgment and using radiology as a complementary tool rather than a primary diagnostic method, healthcare professionals can optimize patient outcomes while fostering essential clinical skills in the next generation of surgeons. As MLDT models continue to evolve, they hold the potential to assist in atypical scenarios, providing faster, clinically-based diagnoses that could further reduce the need for imaging.

6. Current treatment modalities

6.1 Antibiotic-only treatment (conservative management)

The conservative management of appendicitis in children, using antibiotics as an alternative to traditional surgery, has gained increasing attention in recent years. While this approach offers the potential for a less invasive treatment option, it comes with notable challenges, including variable success rates [23] and a considerable risk of treatment failure [24]. These concerns are particularly significant given the anxiety that parents experience when their child's abdominal pain recurs, raising questions about the long-term efficacy and safety of non-operative management [24].

The reported success rates range from 60 to 90% [23, 25]. However, this success is based on imaging-based diagnosis rather than histopathology, raising concerns about the validity of these figures, which are likely overestimated. Imaging alone may not accurately distinguish true appendicitis from other conditions, leading to potential false positives and ultimately creating a misleading sense of success.

A critical aspect of successful conservative management is the careful selection of patients. Not all children with appendicitis are suitable candidates for antibiotic-only treatment. It is essential to identify those who are most likely to respond favorably to this approach, thereby minimizing the risk of failure. Key factors in patient selection include the absence of complicating features such as a fecalith, appendiceal mass, or abscess, along with a thorough evaluation of the overall clinical presentation [26].

Imaging studies are crucial in the selection process for treatment, but they come with their own set of challenges. As previously discussed, reliance on imaging carries inherent risks, particularly the potential for treatment delays in centres where 24-hour services or pediatric radiology expertise are not readily available. These delays must be carefully weighed against the risks of postponing surgical intervention, especially in young children who may deteriorate more rapidly. Such postponements can lead to therapy failure, prolonged hospital stays, increased complications, and higher costs.

Despite these concerns, there is a growing belief that antibiotic treatment may be a promising option for a specific subset of children with uncomplicated appendicitis. However, the success of this approach hinges on the establishment of clear clinical criteria that can reliably distinguish patients who are likely to benefit from antibiotics alone. Until such criteria are well-defined and widely accepted, the author believes that conservative management should be approached with caution. The laparoscopic approach remains the gold standard, providing a definitive and well-established treatment with a high success rate, and any alternative strategy must be rigorously evaluated against this benchmark.

Overall, while the conservative management of appendicitis with antibiotics offers an intriguing alternative to surgery, its application should be reserved for carefully selected patients under well-controlled conditions. Further research and clinical trials are needed to refine patient selection criteria and to ensure that this approach can achieve outcomes comparable to those of laparoscopic surgical treatment.

6.2 Laparoscopic appendectomy

Laparoscopic appendectomy remains the gold standard for treating appendicitis in children, offering a well-established, highly effective surgical solution that consistently outperforms conservative management approaches. This minimally invasive technique not only boasts higher success rates but also ensures faster recovery times and lower complication rates compared to antibiotic-only treatment. The widespread availability of laparoscopic technology in modern healthcare settings further solidifies the rationale for upfront surgical intervention, even in complex cases such as those involving an appendicular mass.

One notable advancement in this field is the single-site laparoscopic-assisted appendectomy [27], a technique where both the laparoscope and grasper are introduced through the umbilicus to grasp and exteriorize the appendix, allowing for extracorporeal removal. This approach has gained traction as a safe, efficient, and cost-effective option for managing non-complicated appendicitis. Studies have demonstrated that this method does not increase the risk of wound site infections or other postoperative complications, providing a reassuring safety profile for pediatric patients. By minimizing incisions and reducing operative time, this technique not only enhances cosmetic outcomes but also diminishes postoperative pain and accelerates the return to normal activities, benefits that are particularly valuable in the pediatric population.

The concept of interval appendectomy, commonly employed in adult patients following the resolution of an appendicular abscess or mass, warrants reconsideration in the pediatric context. Unlike adults, children tend to form softer adhesions, which can be more easily managed during initial surgery. Moreover, immediate appendectomy reduces hospital stay and overall complications [28, 29]. In contrast, the interval appendectomy approach involves an initial course of antibiotics, followed by a planned surgical removal of the appendix during a separate admission. This strategy prolongs the overall treatment duration, leading to a longer cumulative hospital stay and increased healthcare costs. Additionally, the need for an operation after failed conservative management during the initial admission can further burden the patient and family. Immediate appendectomy, therefore, not only spares the child from the anxiety and risks associated with delayed surgery but also eliminates the need for upfront drainage procedures under imaging guidance, which are sometimes required when initial antibiotic therapy fails to improve the patient's condition.

Furthermore, the routine use of drains, a practice often borrowed from adult surgical protocols, may not be justified in pediatric patients. In children, the placement of drains can introduce unnecessary discomfort, increase the risk of infection, and prolong hospital stays without a clear benefit. Studies have shown that children generally have a better postoperative course without the use of drains, and the potential complications associated with drainage systems, such as pain, discomfort, and delayed wound healing, outweigh the perceived advantages [30, 31]. It is crucial to reemphasize that pediatric patients have unique anatomical and physiological characteristics, necessitating surgical practices that are specifically tailored to their needs rather than simply adapted from adult care models.

6.3 Enhanced recovery protocols after appendectomy

Enhanced recovery after surgery (ERAS) protocols have increasingly been adopted in pediatric surgery, including after appendectomy, with the goal of accelerating recovery, reducing hospital stays, minimizing opioid use, and promoting an earlier return to normal activities. These protocols are designed to optimize every stage of the surgical experience, from preoperative preparation to postoperative care, and have been shown to deliver significant benefits for children undergoing appendectomy [32, 33].

One of the key components of ERAS protocols is the emphasis on minimizing opioid use. Traditionally, opioid analgesics have been a mainstay of postoperative pain management. However, the recognition of the risks associated with opioid use, including the potential for dependence and adverse side effects such as nausea and constipation, has led to a shift towards multimodal analgesia. This approach combines non-opioid medications, such as acetaminophen and nonsteroidal anti-inflammatory drugs, with regional anesthesia techniques like transversus abdominis plane blocks. The result is effective pain control with reduced or eliminated reliance on opioids, which in turn facilitates a faster recovery and reduces the likelihood of opioid-related complications.

ERAS protocols also advocate for early mobilization and initiation of a regular diet as soon as possible after surgery. This is supported by evidence suggesting that early mobilization not only improves gastrointestinal function but also reduces the risk of postoperative complications, such as deep vein thrombosis and pulmonary issues. Encouraging children to get out of bed and start walking soon after surgery can significantly shorten their hospital stay and promote a quicker return to normal activities.

Recent literature supports the positive impact of ERAS protocols on recovery times. Studies have shown that children who follow these protocols after appendectomy experience shorter hospital stays, often by one to two days, compared to those managed with traditional care approaches. Moreover, the concept of same-day discharge [34], once considered ambitious, is gaining acceptance in cases of uncomplicated appendicitis. Select children who meet specific criteria, such as stable vital signs, adequate pain control with oral analgesics, and the ability to tolerate oral intake, can safely be discharged on the same day of surgery. This practice not only reduces healthcare costs but also allows children to recover in the comfort of their own homes, which has been shown to improve overall patient satisfaction and reduce the emotional stress associated with hospitalization.

The implementation of ERAS protocols is also associated with a reduction in postoperative complications. By standardizing care and focusing on evidence-based practices, ERAS minimizes variability in treatment, leading to more predictable and favorable outcomes. For instance, the reduced need for opioids under these protocols has been linked to a lower incidence of postoperative ileus, a condition that can prolong hospital stays and delay recovery. Additionally, the encouragement of early feeding and mobilization under ERAS protocols has been shown to enhance overall recovery, as these measures are aligned with the body's natural healing processes.

In conclusion, the adoption of enhanced recovery after surgery protocols in the management of pediatric appendicitis represents a significant advancement in surgical care. By focusing on multimodal pain management, early mobilization, and same-day discharge when appropriate, these protocols not only accelerate recovery but also improve the overall quality of care. The benefits, such as shorter hospital stays, reduced opioid use, fewer complications, and quicker return to normal activities, are well-supported by recent literature, making ERAS an invaluable approach in modern pediatric surgical practice.

7. Outcomes and managing complications after laparoscopic appendectomy in children

Laparoscopic appendectomy is widely recognized as the gold standard for treating appendicitis in children. When compared to adults, children generally experience fewer complications following this procedure, which can be attributed to their unique physiological resilience and the rapidity of their healing processes. However, ensuring optimal outcomes necessitates a well-defined diagnostic approach and the prompt recognition of appendicitis, which is crucial for minimizing the risk of complications.

The importance of early diagnosis cannot be overstated. The sooner the diagnosis is confirmed, the more likely it is that complications can be avoided. Literature supports the notion that the complication rate in children is significantly lower compared to older populations when laparoscopic appendectomy is performed in a timely manner. This emphasizes the need for a streamlined diagnostic process that quickly identifies cases requiring surgical intervention, thereby improving outcomes and reducing the likelihood of complications.

One of the relatively rare complications following laparoscopic appendectomy in children is the formation of an intraabdominal abscess or fluid recollection. While such complications can be concerning, the pediatric population tends to respond exceptionally well to conservative management. Evidence suggests that in many cases, antibiotics alone are sufficient to treat intraabdominal abscesses in children, thereby avoiding the need for more invasive procedures like percutaneous drainage. This contrasts with adult management strategies, where drainage is more commonly employed. The ability of children to recover from such complications with less invasive treatment highlights their uniqueness and remarkable capacity for healing.

When surgical intervention is required, the author advocates for laparoscopic exploration and peritoneal lavage rather than the placement of drains. This approach is associated with faster recovery times, reduced postoperative discomfort, and lower pain levels compared to traditional drainage techniques. The benefits of avoiding drain placement include minimizing the risk of secondary infections, reducing the duration of hospital stays, and enhancing overall patient comfort.

Other potential complications following laparoscopic appendectomy in children include wound infections, adhesions, and bowel obstruction. However, these complications are less frequent in children compared to adults, likely due to the less fibrotic nature of their tissues and their enhanced healing capacity. When managing these complications, a conservative approach is often favored, with surgical intervention reserved for cases where non-operative management fails.

In conclusion, the outcomes following laparoscopic appendectomy in children are generally excellent, with a lower incidence of complications compared to older populations. The key to maintaining these positive outcomes lies in early diagnosis and the application of pediatric-specific management strategies. When complications do arise, a conservative approach can often effectively resolve the issue, allowing children to recover rapidly and return to normal activities with minimal disruption.

8. Conclusion

Pediatric appendicitis demands a nuanced approach that recognizes the distinct needs of children while leveraging the strengths of modern technology. By integrating clinical judgment with AI-driven models like AiPAD, healthcare providers can enhance diagnostic accuracy and treatment outcomes. This chapter has highlighted the importance of maintaining a balance between relying on imaging studies and fostering clinical skills, ultimately advocating for a holistic approach that combines the best of both worlds. As we move forward, the continued refinement and application of these tools will be essential in providing the highest standard of care for pediatric patients.

Author details

Anas Shikha[1*] and Asem Kasem[2]

1 Paediatric Surgery Unit, RIPAS Hospital, Bandar Seri Begawan, Brunei

2 Computer Information Systems, Higher Colleges of Technology, UAE

*Address all correspondence to: dr.a.n.shikha@gmail.com

IntechOpen

© 2024 The Author(s). Licensee IntechOpen. This chapter is distributed under the terms of the Creative Commons Attribution License (http://creativecommons.org/licenses/by/4.0), which permits unrestricted use, distribution, and reproduction in any medium, provided the original work is properly cited.

References

[1] Richardsen I, Schöb D, Ulmer T, Steinau G, Neumann U, Klink C, et al. Etiology of appendicitis in children: The role of bacterial and viral pathogens. Journal of Investigative Surgery. 2016;**29**:74-79. DOI: 10.3109/08941939.2015.1065300

[2] Rautio M, Saxén H, Siitonen A, Nikku R, Jousimies-Somer H. Bacteriology of histopathologically defined appendicitis in children. The Pediatric Infectious Disease Journal. 2000;**19**(11):1078-1083. DOI: 10.1097/00006454-200011000-00010

[3] Stringer M. Anatomy of the infant and child. In: Pediatric Surgery. 2020:10-12. DOI: 10.1007/978-3-642-38482-0_5-1

[4] Bansal S, Banever G, Karrer F, Partrick D. Appendicitis in children less than 5 years old: Influence of age on presentation and outcome. American Journal of Surgery. 2012;**204**(6):1031-1035; discussion 1035. DOI: 10.1016/j.amjsurg.2012.10.003

[5] Acheson J, Banerjee J. Management of suspected appendicitis in children. Archives of Disease in Childhood—Education & Practice Edition. 2010;**95**(1):9-13. DOI: 10.1136/adc.2009.168468

[6] Bianchi V, Giambusso M, De Iacob A, Chiarello MM, Brisinda G. Artificial intelligence in the diagnosis and treatment of acute appendicitis: A narrative review. Updates in Surgery. 2024;**76**(3):783-792. DOI: 10.1007/s13304-024-01801-x

[7] Shikha A, Kasem A. The development and validation of artificial intelligence pediatric appendicitis decision-tree for children 0 to 12 years old. European Journal of Pediatric Surgery. 2023;**33**(5):395-402. DOI: 10.1055/a-1946-0157

[8] Debarnot U, Sperduti M, Di Rienzo F, Guillot A. Experts bodies, experts minds: How physical and mental training shape the brain. Frontiers in Human Neuroscience. 2014;**8**:280. DOI: 10.3389/fnhum.2014.00280. Erratum in: Frontiers in Human Neuroscience. 2015;9:47. DOI: 10.3389/fnhum.2015.00047

[9] Shikha A, Kasem A, Han WSP, Wong JHL. AI-augmented clinical decision in paediatric appendicitis: Can an AI-generated model improve trainees' diagnostic capability? European Journal of Pediatrics. 2024;**183**(3):1361-1366. DOI: 10.1007/s00431-023-05390-6

[10] Goldman RD, Carter S, Stephens D, Antoon R, Mounstephen W, Langer JC. Prospective validation of the pediatric appendicitis score. Journal of Pediatrics. 2008;**153**(2):278-282. DOI: 10.1016/j.jpeds.2008.01.033

[11] Pogorelić Z, Rak S, Mrklić I, Jurić I. Prospective validation of Alvarado score and pediatric appendicitis score for the diagnosis of acute appendicitis in children. Pediatric Emergency Care. 2015;**31**(3):164-168. DOI: 10.1097/PEC.0000000000000375

[12] Kulik D, Uleryk E, Maguire J. Does this child have appendicitis? A systematic review of clinical prediction rules for children with acute abdominal pain. Journal of Clinical Epidemiology. 2013;**66**(1):95-104. DOI: 10.1016/j.jclinepi.2012.09.004

[13] Stone M. Cross-validatory choice and assessment of statistical predictions.

Journal of the Royal Statistical Society: Series B (Methodological). 1974;**36**(2):111-133. DOI: 10.1111/j.2517-6161.1974.tb00994.x

[14] Martin A, Vollman D, Adler B, Caniano D. CT scans may not reduce the negative appendectomy rate in children. Journal of Pediatric Surgery. 2004;**39**(6):886-890; discussion 886-890. DOI: 10.1016/j.jpedsurg.2004.02.034

[15] Miano DI, Silvis RM, Popp JM, Culbertson MC, Campbell B, Smith SR. Abdominal CT does not improve outcome for children with suspected acute appendicitis. The Western Journal of Emergency Medicine. 2015;**16**(7):974-982. DOI: 10.5811/westjem.2015.10.25576

[16] Baykara A. Acute appendicitis in children: Evaluation of the diagnostic efficacy of ultrasonography and computed tomography. Cureus. 2023;**15**(8):e43860. DOI: 10.7759/cureus.43860

[17] Keating E, Orth R, Bisset G, Starke H, Cruz A. Utility of computed tomography overreading and abdominal ultrasound in children with suspected appendicitis and nondiagnostic computed tomography at community hospitals. Pediatric Emergency Care. 2020;**36**(12):564-570. DOI: 10.1097/PEC.0000000000002283

[18] Estey A, Poonai N, Lim R. Appendix not seen: The predictive value of secondary inflammatory sonographic signs. Pediatric Emergency Care. 2013;**29**(4):435-439. DOI: 10.1097/pec.0b013e318289e8d5

[19] Schuh S, Man C, Cheng A, et al. Predictors of non-diagnostic ultrasound scanning in children with suspected appendicitis. Journal of Pediatrics. 2011;**158**(1):112-118. DOI: 10.1016/j.jpeds.2010.07.035

[20] Brenner DJ, Hall EJ. Computed tomography—An increasing source of radiation exposure. New England Journal of Medicine. 2007;**357**(22):2277-2284. DOI: 10.1056/nejmra072149

[21] Brody AS, Frush DP, Huda W, et al. Radiation risk to children from computed tomography. Pediatrics. 2007;**120**(3):677-682. DOI: 10.1542/peds.2007-1910

[22] Pearce MS, Salotti JA, Little MP, et al. Radiation exposure from CT scans in childhood and subsequent risk of leukaemia and brain tumours: A retrospective cohort study. The Lancet. 2012;**380**(9840):499-505. DOI: 10.1016/s0140-6736(12)60815-0

[23] Xu J, Adams S, Liu Y, Karpelowsky J. Nonoperative management in children with early acute appendicitis: A systematic review. Journal of Pediatric Surgery. 2017;**52**(9):1409-1415. DOI: 10.1016/j.jpedsurg.2017.05.003

[24] Lipsett SC, Monuteaux MC, Shanahan KH, Bachur RG. Nonoperative management of uncomplicated appendicitis. Pediatrics. 2022;**149**(5):e2021054693. DOI: 10.1542/peds.2021-054693

[25] Bethell GS, Rees CM, Sutcliffe J, Hall NJ. Outcomes one year after non-operative management of uncomplicated appendicitis in children: Children with appendicitis during the coronavirus pandemic (CASCADE) study. BJS Open. 2023;7:zrad055. DOI: 10.1093/bjsopen/zrad055

[26] Huang L, Yin Y, Yang L, Wang C, Li Y, Zhou Z. Comparison of antibiotic therapy and appendectomy for acute uncomplicated appendicitis in children: A meta-analysis. JAMA Pediatrics. 2017;**171**(5):426-434. DOI: 10.1001/jamapediatrics.2017.0057

[27] Perea L, Peranteau WH, Laje P. Transumbilical extracorporeal laparoscopic-assisted appendectomy. Journal of Pediatric Surgery. 2018;**53**(2):256-259. DOI: 10.1016/j.jpedsurg.2017.11.012

[28] Das BB, Nayak KN, Mohanty SK, Sahoo AK. A retrospective analysis of conservative management versus early surgical intervention in appendicular lump. Cureus. 2022;**14**(1):e21784. DOI: 10.7759/cureus.21784

[29] Samuel M, Hosie G, Holmes K. Prospective evaluation of nonsurgical versus surgical management of appendiceal mass. Journal of Pediatric Surgery. 2002;**37**(6):882-886. DOI: 10.1053/jpsu.200

[30] Neville JJ, Aldeiri B. Drain placement in paediatric complicated appendicitis: A systematic review and meta-analysis. Pediatric Surgery International. 2023;**39**(1):171. DOI: 10.1007/s00383-023-05457-3

[31] Tran HV, Quang HV, Long DT, The HC, Dang CP, Chen MK, et al. Laparoscopic treatment of appendiceal peritonitis without drainage in children—A prospective randomized clinical trial. Journal of Pediatric Surgery Open. 2023;**15**:100046. DOI: 10.1016/j.yjpso.2023.100046

[32] Zhang JG, Li HW, Wu XM, Yu HB, Liu YH, Qi L, et al. The impact of enhanced recovery after surgery on inflammatory indicators and prognosis related to complex appendicitis in children. Frontiers in Pediatrics. 2023;**11**:1261191. DOI: 10.3389/fped.2023.1261191

[33] Al-Taher R, Alshahwan H, Abdelhadi S, Abeeleh FA, Rashdan M, Amarin M, et al. Enhanced recovery concepts in paediatric patients who underwent appendectomy: A retrospective cohort study at a tertiary university hospital. The Journal of International Medical Research. 2023;**51**(2):3000605231158524. DOI: 10.1177/03000605231158524

[34] Lo HYA, Yang C, Rettig RL, Chung J, Shaul D, Sydorak R. Same day discharge after pediatric laparoscopic appendectomy in community hospitals. Journal of Pediatric Surgery. 2022;**57**(7):1242-1248. DOI: 10.1016/j.jpedsurg.2022.02.038